REMEDIATION OF THE

Struggling Medical Learner

REMEDIATION OF THE

Struggling Medical Learner

Jeannette Guerrasio, MD

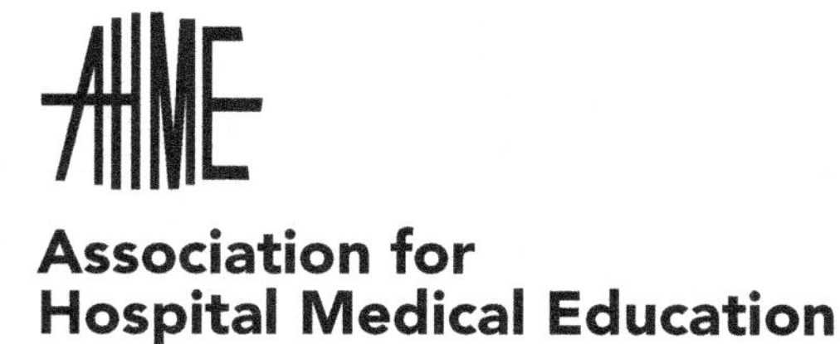

All primary study data presented by Dr. Guerrasio has been collected in accordance with, and approved by, the Colorado Multiple Institutional Review Board.

The case examples are either invented or are amalgams of real cases in which names and all identifying information have been changed.

Association for Hospital Medical Education
109 Brush Creek Road
Irwin, PA 15642
(724) 864-7321 Phone
(724) 864-6153 Fax
info@ahme.org Email
www.ahme.org

ISBN 978-0-615-80058-5
Library of Congress Control Number: 2013939502

Cover and Interior design by AllyB Design, LLC.
allybdesign@yahoo.com

Printed in the United States of America by Lightning Source, LaVergne, Tennessee

Foreword

Medical education is not a career for the faint of heart. Society expects and deserves optimal performance from physicians. Those of us engaged in training them are all too aware that it is a highly flawed enterprise. Medical training is a complex, long term, costly undertaking. The stakes are high and our ability to accurately assess our success or failure is sorrowfully limited. Because of this we must invest in developing the judgment and skills of front line medical educators to identify and remediate our students and residents who aren't meeting high standards. This means that responsibility for remediation should be part of every medical educator's job description. And yet, in my experience, only a few take up this challenge with the intelligence, passion, compassion and enthusiasm required to be successful. Jeannette Guerrasio is such a physician educator and her keenness for the subject and respect for the struggling learner is what makes this book required reading for all medical educators.

Like Guerrasio, I find working with struggling students intellectually and personally challenging, satisfying and meaningful. Trainees are often deeply grateful when given the opportunity to address a vexing weakness in a supportive and confidential manner. Even when the outcome is not ideal for the student, the remediation process can be clarifying and satisfying. And yet, many of my colleagues do not share my optimism. And I understand why. Even I, when faced with a student, resident or colleague who is flailing, have that "heart sink" feeling. It is difficult to work with a trainee who "doesn't get it" or "can't do it." This presents not only an intellectual but also an emotional challenge. Initially, some of us might blame the student for being weak or the system for allowing such a trainee to get this far. Some of us prefer to steer clear of confrontation in general. Many of us identify and empathize with the students and feel tender to them and protective of their feelings. There are those of us who are convinced that someone else, anyone else, should take responsibility for addressing a struggling learner. For whatever reason, more often than is right, we abdicate our responsibility and fail to identify our struggling students early, therefore ensuring that they do not get help. So let's agree now that this is not justifiable given our social contract with society and the privilege we are granted as a profession to self-regulate.

I believe that many of us avoid intervening because we aren't fully convinced that effective, practical remediation strategies exist. This is why Guerrasio's book, *Remediation of the Struggling Medical Learner* is likely to become a foundational text for faculty development in health profession education. This gem of a book is written in a clear, direct style. It is peppered with illustrative examples and sage advice. Individual chapters can easily be the basis for a "brown bag" lunch series to onboard new inpatient attendings or ambulatory preceptors. In this volume she synthesizes, for the first time, what is known about remediation of medical competence and proposes a practical and evidence-based approach to remediation.

Physicians are uniquely qualified to conduct remediation since we are trained to deal with complex problems in uncertain, chaotic, high-stakes circumstances. We have a diagnostic, prognostic, and therapeutic model which serves the tasks of remediation well, and are expert at combining highly rigorous, analytic critical thinking to complex problems with skillful, respectful and compassionate communication. We have a culture of respecting confidentiality and attending to complicated ethical concerns, and, most importantly, we fulfill an important obligation to our profession and our patients when we effectively take on this responsibility.

All medical schools should have their own high profile, well-resourced, physician-led, remediation program, modeled after the one Guerrasio describes in this book. The existence of such a program communicates to the community, trainees and faculty two important things. First, that learners who struggle will get the respectful and effective help they need and deserve. And second, that as a profession we have the courage and conviction needed to ensure that all physicians will be fully supported to meet society's highest standards.

Adina Kalet, MD, MPH
Gold Professor of Humanism and Professionalism
Director of the Program for Professional Development
Assessment and Outcomes, Office of Medical Education
New York University School of Medicine

Preface

While all medical training programs, from undergraduate to graduate medical education, struggle with underperforming learners, the number of resources available to teaching faculty and course and program directors is insufficient. This book, *Remediation of the Struggling Medical Learner*, was written based on the literature as well as my years of experience working with learners in need of remedial teaching.

By consolidating information and organizing the content according to the way clinicians are trained to solve problems, this text offers a practical approach within a format that is easy to read. Real life examples of struggling learners and genuine faculty reactions illustrate the guidelines for working with these students.

Remediation of the Struggling Medical Learner was written to provide a structure for the identification of the underperforming medical learner, a familiar framework for the diagnosis of learner difficulties and a step-by-step approach for the remediation of the most common and most challenging learner deficiencies.

Since giving feedback is both an extremely difficult skill to master and essential to remediation, one section is devoted to how to give feedback and is specifically designed for those working with learners who have fallen behind.

Given that many medical schools, residency programs and fellowship programs do not have formal remediation policies and procedures, this book also provides institutional and faculty guidance on how to build and sustain a remediation program.

The phrase "medical learners" was chosen because it encompasses the levels of medical training from student through residents and fellows. In addition, the content of the text is applicable to other health care professionals, including nurse practitioners and physician assistants.

I have addressed you, the reader, directly in this book and have taken some grammatical liberties that more accurately reflect what we would say in conversation rather than what we would write in a formal document. I welcome your feedback on the book and hope it encourages your interest in this growing field. If you wish to share your thoughts about *Remediation of the Struggling Medical Learner* and/or are interested in collaborating on multi-institution studies related to research on remediation, please email me: Jeannette.Guerrasio@ucdenver.edu.

Wishing you and your learners great success,

Jeannette Guerrasio, MD

Acknowledgements

My sincerest thank you to my mentor, Eva Aagaard, MD, who has supported my professional development and my interest in building a remediation program, and helped me to open many new doors; Suzanne Brandenburg, MD, Maureen Garrity, PhD, and Carol Rumack, MD, who have provided opportunities working with their medical learners and helping me navigate the world of academia; my friend, poet and editor Max Regan, MFA, for his honest feedback, availability and encouragement; my copy editors Lisa Birman, MFA, and Catherine (Carrie) Eckart, MBA, for their detailed and invaluable proofreading; my dear friend Ethan Cumbler, MD, for his brilliant ideas and support; and my partner Deborah Lehman, MD, who has endured my absence while working and who has been endlessly supportive.

With much gratitude, I wish to thank my literary agent, Joan Parker from Parker Literary Agency, LLC, who has worked tirelessly to guide me through the publication process and to find the perfect academic society to represent this work. Thanks to the support of the Association for Hospital Medical Education (AHME), AHME Executive Director Kimball Mohn, MD and Lightning Source, I have the opportunity to share with others what I have learned about medical learner remediation over the years. Lastly, I would like to recognize AllyB Design, LLC for their graphic designs, including the covers, tables and figures and final revisions. I am very lucky to have found such a productive and collaborative team of truly great people.

Table of Contents

SECTION 1:

Introduction to the Identification, Diagnosis and Remediation of the Struggling Medical Learner

The task of the excellent teacher is to stimulate "apparently ordinary" people to unusual effort. The tough problem is not in identifying winners: it is in making winners out of ordinary people.

K. Patricia Cross*

*From Parnell, Dale. The Neglected Majority. Washington, DC: The Community College Press.1985.

CHAPTER 1:

The Need for Remediation

Dr. Miller spent 4 hours tossing and turning in bed. He finally sat up, put on his slippers, and walked to the foyer closet. Distracted, he pulled on his winter coat, wrapped a scarf around his neck, and tossed on a hat and gloves. Dr. Miller stepped out into the crisp night air, so cold it briefly took his breath away. Walking alone in the darkness of night seemed to help clear his mind. Tomorrow, he would find out if he would lose his medical license.

The state medical board had reviewed him 5 times since he graduated from residency just 3 years ago. Most recently, he gave a woman in septic shock the diuretic furosemide. She was infected with pneumonia and hypotensive, but her history of congestive heart failure, from left ventricular dysfunction, threw him off course. He anchored on the patient's history and his vague memories of the Starling Curve, despite a physical exam that supported her dehydration. There was no jugular venous distension, no edema, no S3 heart sound and she was warm. His clinical reasoning had failed him...again. She died and he could only anticipate another lawsuit. He was already facing 2 malpractice suits, which his lawyers and malpractice insurance company promised he would lose if he didn't settle.

Dr. Miller was consumed with guilt, regret and frustration. During his non-clinical years in medical school, he did very well, acing every exam. During the clinical years, he was a quiet student and his assumed "shyness" hid his deficits well. But by the end of his third year of medical school, he silently knew that he was struggling. He wanted to ask for help, but didn't know where to turn or whom he could trust. His fourth year grades and evaluations were marginal, but he had already matched into a competitive residency and graduation was guaranteed.

All through residency, he received borderline evaluations. His quiet persona helped him slide under the radar the first 2 years and he was so likeable that his colleagues often helped to the point of making his decisions for him. He lacked clinical reasoning skills. It wasn't until he was paired with a weak intern in December of his third year that his deficits could no longer be ignored...or could they?

He received an honest and scathing evaluation from his supervising attending, claiming that he was a danger to patients and not ready to graduate. The residency program director panicked. They had been unsuccessful at remediation in the past, and few faculty had the time, dedication and skills to mentor this failing resident; however, he only had 2 more challenging rotations left in his residency. For both, he was intentionally paired with the strongest intern to ensure the safety of the patients. With a strong intern, the patients received good care and the evaluators assumed that Dr. Miller was a capable physician and the primary decision maker for the patients' care. Dr. Miller received 2 strong evaluations for these challenging rotations.

The residency program director did not think that he should graduate, but feared the costs and hassles of litigation. The lawyers at the university warned that there was not a solid trail of documentation highlighting his deficits, and in fact, only one faculty member recorded his concerns. The resident could argue that he was evaluated unfairly or that the attending was prejudiced against him. The residency program director felt obligated to graduate him with only one weak evaluation in his file.

Instead of pacing the neighborhood, in the shadow of darkness, his life could have been different. What if an individualized learning plan had been created for him in his third year of medical school when he first struggled? What if his residency program had a remediation program in place to work with him? Would it have saved his career? His patients? His pride? Would he have chosen a different specialty or career better suited to his skills?

From the beginning

All medical learners struggle at some point along their educational journey. While the type and degree of struggle varies, it is our role as teachers to help all of our learners reach their maximum potential. In speaking with medical training program directors across the country, it quickly became apparent that most training programs and teachers struggle with underperforming learners and are seeking guidance on an individual and institutional level on how to help this population of learners. Yet, teachers have very little guidance on how to remediate struggling medical learners. The published literature on remediation in medical education is minimal and there are no concise texts to guide program and course directors, institutions, teachers or struggling learners themselves.

At the University of Colorado, I, with the support and mentorship of the Vice Chair of Education Eva Aagaard, MD, created and built a remediation program for struggling medical learners. Initially, the program was developed based on the limited information available in the literature and the experience of senior teachers and educators at a variety of institutions. I was also inspired and guided by the work of Jeffrey Weise, MD at the University of California, San Francisco, where the remediation program COUGAR (A Curriculum to Observe Underperformers and Give Assisted Remediation) was developed. With each case, I continued to adapt and build a remediation program with strategies based on my experience working with struggling learners, their feedback on the program, my understanding of the system of medical education and the needs of the university leadership. While the program was first created to help struggling residents, it was extremely well received and expanded to include medical students who performed poorly on their internal medicine clerkship. The program continued to grow as word spread campus-wide of the academic success of the participants, the appreciated need of such a program and the administrative and legal support it provided. The inclusion of students, residents, fellows and faculty learners has only added to my experience in total number of cases, as well as giving me a broader perspective on the educational needs of learners across the education continuum.

Based on collective experience, this book was written to provide a practical structure for the identification of the struggling medical learner, a familiar framework for the diagnosis of the learner's deficit(s) and a step-by-step approach for the remediation of the most common and encompassing learner deficiencies. Program, clerkship and course directors, teaching faculty and learners themselves can use the concepts and models effectively. Since most medical schools and residency and fellowship programs do not have formalized remediation programs, the book also provides institutional and faculty guidance on how to build and sustain a remediation program. Finally, a chapter on giving feedback is included because it is extremely difficult to give corrective feedback and it is essential to remediation. This section provides practical advice and examples of how to give feedback, with tips specifically designed for those working with struggling medical learners.

This problem of the struggling medical learner impacts the education and professional success of medical students, residents, fellows, attending physicians and other clinicians. After extensive discussions with teachers across the fields of medicine, I grew to appreciate the overlap and commonalities across all disciplines of medical education. I have chosen to use the words "medical learners" because it encompasses the levels of allopathic and osteopathic medical training from student through attending physician. In addition, the text is likely just as applicable to training of nurse practitioners and physician assistants, their educational programs and faculty, and to select physical therapy programs.

Teaching those who need us most

Working with medical learners is a tremendous honor, opportunity and responsibility. Most of our learners demonstrate professional and personal growth throughout their training programs and by graduation have acquired the skills necessary to be competent practitioners of medicine. A small percentage, however, do not thrive or find success in the standard methods of medical training. Do you get a pit in your stomach when you hear that one of your learners is struggling? Do you feel overwhelmed or discouraged? With a standardized, successful approach to the learner in difficulty, the task of remediation still requires time and energy, but can be approached with focus, confidence and hope. Struggling learners who require remediation and individualized learning plans challenge our true skills and abilities as teachers. While it is easy to teach and mentor the learners who, in truth, would succeed in any environment, the struggling learners differentiate the quality teachers from their peers.

When a learner is struggling in the midst of his or her education, a remediation strategy is necessary. In colloquial language, remediation is the correction of an underlying deficit. The American Board of Internal Medicine's Chief Residents' Workshop on Problem Residents defined a medical learner in need of remediation as a "trainee who demonstrates a significant enough problem that requires intervention by someone of authority, usually the program director or chief resident." In 1998, Vaughn, et al. published, "The Problem Learner" in which they defined a struggling learner as "a learner whose academic performance is significantly below performance potential because of a specific affective, cognitive, structural or interpersonal difficulty."

While remediation often has a negative connotation reserved for the failing student, I challenge you to broaden your perspective. All students and practitioners have areas of weakness, as they have areas of strength. Remediation is teaching that is individualized and targeted towards these areas of weakness to maximize the learner's potential. We would all benefit from this customized form of remediation. Many techniques in this text will improve your skills as a teacher of all learners of all abilities, including yourself as a lifelong self-directed learner.

Just how many learners need remediation?

My inbox seemed to be overflowing as I received 4 emails today voicing concerns about 4 different learners. Only one had been referred before. Jack is a resident, failing to pay attention to details in clinic and has been resistant to getting treatment for his depression. Then there is a student, Maria, who passed her clerkship but can't write an H&P, and the fellow, Dimitry who failed his specialty boards. Not to mention Isaac, the resident who fought with his attending in front of a family. The feelings are always mixed; sadness for the struggling learner, disappointment for the multiple uphill battles that lie ahead and excitement that perhaps the program can truly improve the trajectory of someone's career. How many more will be sent my way this week? Just how many learners are struggling?

Medical student clinical clerkship directors throughout the United States seek to remediate medical students who do not meet the standards of their institutions or who have other deficits that prevent them from becoming safe and independent residents. Up to 15% of third year medical students struggle during their clerkships, and up to 11% struggle during the fourth year. Unfortunately, teachers and course directors should expect these numbers to increase. One should anticipate both an absolute rise in the number of struggling students as medical school classes grow, as well as a rise in the percentage needing remediation as admission requirements change to expand recruitment and class size.

A national survey of Internal Medicine Residency program directors conducted by Yao and Wright in 2000 demonstrated a point prevalence of residents in need of remediation of 7%, while the American Board of Internal Medicine estimates that 8 to 15% of residents have significant areas of learner difficulty. These statistics vary little from one specialty to the next, with the exception of General Surgery which has reported that up to 1/3 of their residents need remediation. Some physicians hope that the problem will just go away, but ignoring the impact and challenge of the underperforming learners has devastating consequences. In fact, the percentage of residents in difficulty has grown at the same frequency for the past several decades and, as with struggling medical students, the number of struggling residents is only expected to grow as the number of total residency positions available increases. This is compounded by the fact that residents are expected to maintain the same level of proficiency despite declining patient encounters and work hours during training.

Consider this: the prevalence of struggling medical students is approximately the same as the prevalence of struggling residents. Does this reflect the concern that deficiencies do not resolve without meaningful intervention? When asked, 17% of practicing physicians reported that they were aware of and had encountered an impaired or incompetent colleague within the past 3 years. Deficiencies in medicine are observed across multiple levels of training, from students through practicing attendings. Does this imply that physician trainees are not the only medical learners who struggle? Are there strugglers among all levels and types of medical learners? Fortunately, the principles of remediation are universal and even apply to physicians who are competent but want to be better.

Despite the magnitude of the problem, we as teachers and educators struggle to rapidly identify, accurately diagnose and adequately remediate medical learners. An extensive literature review on the subject identifies many deficits and limits to the development of remediation programs. To begin, methods for identifying learners with deficiencies are not standardized and, until this text, readily available strategies for remediation were not compiled in one resource. In reviewing individual journal articles you will find that there is a paucity of data on reliable, valid, practical assessment tools. While a few well-designed studies exist, they are small and only single institution studies. In total, searches for remediation guidelines demonstrate the overwhelming lack of evidence to guide best practices in remediation.

Why invest the time, money and people power?

It is Friday morning and I have 2 new learners to meet with. I know that the sooner I meet with them, the quicker they can begin remediation and correct their bad habits before they become engrained, and before they fail again. I flip open my calendar and, just as I thought, I am scheduled from at least 7 to 5 for the next 3 weeks. In truth, I do have 3 days free, clearly marked as "days off." Do I cancel existing meetings, extend my workday or come in on my days off? The inconvenience that changing my schedule or extending my hours would cause pales in comparison to the impact that our meetings may have. It also reminds me to role model the level of professionalism that I expect of my learners when they are caring for patients. I choose to come in on my day off, Memorial Day, when the residents are available.

Helping our struggling medical learners is crucially important. If you have ever worked with a failing learner, or even a learner who is performing just below average, you would have noticed that it takes much more time. You, the learner and the other members of the clinical team spend extra time teaching, correcting the learner's mistakes in understanding and practice, supervising and providing structure needed to guide the learner's performance. And while we all have good intentions when it comes to teaching weaker learners, it can be exhausting, challenging, unpleasant and unsatisfying. You may end up spending as much time preserving the morale of the team and his classmates as you do working with the struggling learner. From a program director and administrative perspective, struggling students and poor morale impact the reputation of your program and institution and affect recruitment.

TABLE 1.1 Importance of Medical Learner Remediation

1. Struggling learners take up time
2. Ignoring it affects morale of health care team and learner's peers
3. Can impact program's reputation
4. Deficiencies don't resolve without intervention
5. Lack of remediation impacts patient safety and quality of care
6. Our obligation is to educate all learners

There are several more fundamental reasons to be invested in remediation of our weaker medical learners. First, the deficiencies often do not resolve without intervention. Second, these learners impact patient satisfaction, patient safety, and quality of care. Third, it is our *obligation* to teach *all* of our learners, not just the ones who are easy to teach, more enjoyable to teach or those who can teach themselves. The best teachers are truly distinguished not by their ability to teach the brightest and quickest, but by their ability to teach and connect with all of their students (**Table 1.1**). The last reason is self-monitoring.

Self-monitoring

It is our responsibility to self-monitor our profession. Self-monitoring our profession requires a high degree of ethical investment and commitment that supersedes our own discomfort and fear of confronting others and resistance to giving critical and corrective feedback. We must dedicate time and energy to self-monitoring. No other group of individuals is better qualified to assess and monitor the performance of our learners and soon to be peers. We must preserve the integrity of our profession by diligently teaching, accurately evaluating and providing remediation for our future and current colleagues. At the end of the day, I want to know that I could willingly and confidently sign my patients out to my learners or have them take care of my own family members.

There is currently a national movement to improve the quality of patient care, from systems improvements to the patient-centered medical home. Let us not leave out a concentrated effort to improve the competency of our medical providers. Be a pioneer at your institution. You can create a program and/or a culture that supports the success of struggling learners and thereby improves the educational experience for all learners.

The subsequent sections and chapters will examine common deficits among medical learners and explore how struggling learners are identified. I will go on to provide a framework for diagnosing the medical learner's deficiency(ies), determining the level of deficiency and identifying the responsibility of the evaluators.

CHAPTER 2:

Introduction to Identification and Diagnosis

Sasha comes to my office teary with bloodshot eyes, looking down at her feet, as if lost in a forest. She thought that she had been doing well on her first clinical rotation of medical school. She can't remember ever getting negative feedback or being told she had done something incorrectly; yet, she received a failing score for her oral presentation skills. I hand her my tissue box, which I had just replenished. "I'm Dr. Guerrasio," I say softly, "and I think I can help, but first I need to know more. Can I ask you a few questions?"

Help-avoidance behaviors are indirectly related to academic outcomes and negatively correlated with medical school grade point average and clinical performance. Even after failing, only 50% of medical students will seek help. Since learners will not seek help, we must find them early and direct them towards a more productive path.

As teachers and evaluators we must begin by learning to identify strengths and weaknesses in our students for the purposes of both identifying underperforming learners and diagnosing their area(s) of difficulty. You will also find that these skills will help you to better assess all of your learners, allow you to provide more thoughtful, specific and useful feedback and to write more accurate and thorough evaluations and letters of recommendation.

Although limited, there is some data in the literature on struggling medical learners at various stages of training. In 1999, PJ Olmesdahl found that the most serious concerns of second and third year medical students were related to volume of work, learning methods and strategies, time management and inadequate study time. This was further categorized in 2009 by G Paul et al. through a survey of medical schools, where she found the most common problems across all four years of training to be:

- Organizing large amounts of information
- Integrating large amounts of information
- Time Management

- Test taking
- Test anxiety
- Stress or anxiety not associated with testing

As you might have anticipated based on your own experience with failing learners, the most common deficits vary based on level of training. Much of our data regarding struggling residents comes from a national survey of Internal Medicine Residency program directors, conducted by Yao and Wright that was published in 2000. Their study identified the following deficiencies from most to least common:

- Insufficient medical knowledge
- Poor clinical judgment
- Inefficient use of time
- Inappropriate interactions with colleagues or staff
- Provision of poor or inadequate medical care to patients
- Unsatisfactory clinical skills
- Unsatisfactory humanistic behaviors with patients
- Excessive or unexplained tardiness or absences
- Unacceptable moral or ethical behaviors

At the University of Colorado from 2006–2011, the following learner deficits were identified across the education continuum (see **Figure 2.1**). Our data reflects that the most common medical student deficits are medical knowledge, clinical reasoning and judgment, communication and mental well-being. The term mental well-being was chosen to encompass psychosocial stressors and psychiatric diagnoses, including substance abuse and learning disabilities.

As learners progress through training into practice, it appears that deficits in communication, medical knowledge and mental well-being become less frequent, while the prevalence of poor professionalism and poor clinical reasoning and judgment increases. This may reflect the need to pass all required medical knowledge exams and maintain a benchmark of mental well-being prior to graduating from medical school. The United States Medical Licensing Exam's (USMLE) Step 2 Clinical skills portion also helps to ensure minimal competence in communication skills (see **Table 2.1**).

The increased percentage of communication deficits among the student population may reflect their limited life and clinical experience. Perhaps the students with poor communication skills have been weeded out prior to reaching higher levels of training and, therefore, this deficit is seen at lower frequency among attendings. It is also possible that dramatic cultural changes

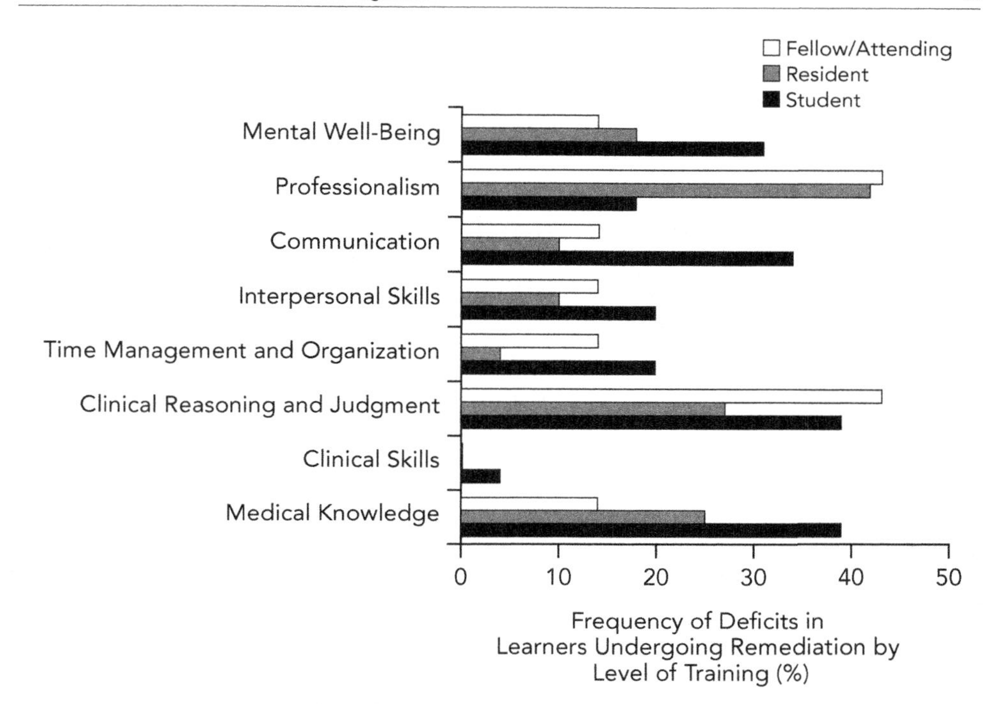

FIGURE 2.1 Frequency of Deficits in Learners Undergoing Remediation by Level of Training. The data includes 68 residents, 51 medical students and 7 fellows/attendings, 58% of whom identify as male. You will notice that the identified deficits change with level of training and that most of the learners have multiple deficits. The average number of deficits is 1.6; 1.9 for medical students, 1.4 for residents and 1.6 for fellows/attendings.

TABLE 2.1 Deficits Among Medical Learners by Stage. The table summarizes the data collected at various institutions over various levels of training in the past 15 years.

Early Learners	Advanced Learners
Medical Knowledge	Professionalism
Clinical Reasoning—integration of data	Clinical Judgment—decision making
	Time Management and Organization
Time Management and Organization	Interpersonal Skills
Communication	
Mental Well-being	

in communication styles are reflected in this data. Modes of social networking and media culture communication, including texting and computer networking, may greatly affect students' communication skills in a way that may not impact more senior residents and attendings.

Identification, the First Hurdle

In the remediation of our most challenged learners, identification is the first of many obstacles to be overcome. There are early and late identifiers that a learner has fallen behind and there are various modes by which faculty, residents and students can notify clerkship, course or program directors of his or her concerns.

Early in a course, you may hear verbal comments about a learner's poor performance from supervising faculty, chiefs, residents, students, nursing staff, patients, administrative assistants or (rarely) the individual learner (see **Table 2.2**). Perhaps your institution has a system for early reporting of concerns. Do you have a mechanism in place for early reporting of struggling learners that goes directly to the director and occurs prior to the evaluation? Have you used this reporting system or written to your course director to voice concerns? If you are the course director, are you receiving notification of weak learners early enough? Many institutions have reporter initiated reporting systems that go to

TABLE 2.2 Common Identifiers of Struggling Learners

Early
Verbal comments by faculty, chiefs, residents, nurses, students, administrative assistants, peers, learner himself/herself
Reporting system for general concerns
Critical incident or patient safety reports
Mid-clerkship clinical performance evaluations
Simulations, OSCEs, CEX or mini-CEX
Late
Written examinations
Clinical performance examinations
Formal evaluations of competencies/professionalism
Peer or global multi-source assessments
During group review or grading session
Course Failure

specific committees, course directors or attendings. These systems, however, are often limited to problems related to professionalism or patient safety. Tragically, when systems of early identification and notification fail, some struggling learners are identified only after a critical incident has occurred.

Formalized and required mid-course clinical performance evaluations may be helpful in identifying struggling learners before it is too late and also in cueing the teacher to provide mid-rotation feedback to the learner. These evaluations give the learner information about her/his performance: what s/he is doing successfully that s/he should continue to do; what s/he is doing wrong that s/he should stop doing; and what s/he should change to improve her/his overall performance. If the evaluation is received mid-course, then s/he still has time to demonstrate that s/he can incorporate constructive criticism and improve her/his performance before a course grade is assigned.

Other modes of evaluation may also be used mid-course to identify learner deficits. Consider how simulation, observed clinical examinations of either a full H&P or a focused encounter (CEX or mini-CEX) or objective structured clinical examinations (OSCE) may be incorporated to improve mid-course feedback and allow for individualization of curriculum as needed.

Although late notification is helpful for the learner in his overall education and for subsequent courses, it often comes too late to impact the grades and evaluations of the current rotation. It also doesn't allow the learner to work in the same environment to improve based on the information received. For example, if a student's evaluation demonstrates deficiencies in performing the newborn exam and the student does not have any more rotations working with neonates, it will be much more difficult to provide the student with opportunities to work on these skills. Some examples of late identifiers include end-of-course written examinations, clinical performance exams, formal evaluations of competency, peer or global multi-source (formally known as 360°) assessments and a group review or grading session. Sometimes the first notification may be a course failure.

Take a moment to reflect on your own institution. Do you know what policies and modes of notification are in place when you identify a struggling learner or someone comes to you with concerns? Are there ways of improving the current system to include some of the items in Table 2.2? Does your institution use other means that I have not specifically addressed? If your institution has a system in place, is it used in a timely fashion to maximize its effectiveness for the learner, or is the information received or reviewed too late to truly impact learner performance?

Other barriers

Unfortunately, timing is not the only barrier to identification. There is a lack of willingness on the part of evaluators to report or record negative evaluations for many reasons. There are fears of repercussions, anticipation of an appeals process and/or lack of investment in remediation. Academic faculty promotions are to some degree dependent on the evaluations received from learners and faculty therefore feel the need to ensure positive reciprocal feelings from their learners. Faculty also cite lack of knowledge of what to specifically document, lack of remediation options and fear regarding their level of personal responsibility to provide remediation. Evaluating faculty also state that the reason that they do not report struggling learners is that they lack the ability or knowledge to use the grading system, question their ability to fairly and fully assess a problem and fear causing unnecessary harm as the standards are not well defined.

These barriers require a cultural change, respect for the missions of the educational program and trust in the system. It requires trust that the information relayed will be used to educate and benefit the student, rather than being purely punitive or simply ignored. A well-built system and approach will lead to confidence in your remediation efforts and willingness on the part of teachers and learners to participate and contribute to the program. Once the program has been established and the culture changes, many of the referrals and concerns will come unsolicited, readily and in volume.

There are also learner-focused barriers. Is the quiet student just shy or is he quietly masking deficits and flying under the radar? How much of the learner's performance is his rather than the contributions from other team members or consultants? What about the learner who is secretly working 100 hours/week just to keep up with his peers? Identification requires an astute investigation by an evaluator and diagnostician who pays attention to all of the details and doesn't let their learners hide behind others or themselves.

CHAPTER 3:

Framework for Diagnosing Area of Learner Difficulty

I just made myself a cup of tea in preparation for the work that lies ahead. I settle into my desk chair to review a stack of student evaluations. The scores and comments on the first 2 students are stellar; however, the comments on Addison's evaluation say, "Her oral presentations are poor and she is far behind her peers. Recommend that she practices more." Hmm, I think, she has a problem with presenting cases but that could mean a medical knowledge, clinical reasoning, organization and/or communication problem. I need more information before I can create a remediation plan.

Just as frameworks are used in clinical medicine, a framework is necessary for diagnosing a learner's deficit(s). When an underperforming student is brought to your attention, via verbal comments, written performance evaluations, and/or written or clinical performance examinations, approach the concern as you would in clinical medicine—start with a differential diagnosis.

The Accreditation Council for Graduate Medical Education (ACGME) published the Outcome Project in 1999 to standardize the assessment of residents by establishing a list of 6 competencies that all physicians are required to demonstrate prior to graduating from residency and in the context of their specialties. The 6 competencies are: medical knowledge; patient care; interpersonal skills and communication; professionalism; practice-based learning and improvement; and systems-based practice (see **Table 3.1**). While the competencies of medical knowledge, patient care, interpersonal skills, and professionalism are already familiar to medical educators, the concepts of practice-based learning and improvement as well as systems-based practice have been introduced more recently and it may be helpful to specifically define these competencies. Specifically, competence in practice-based learning and improvement requires that a resident self-assess her/his strengths and weaknesses, identify her/his limits, set new learning and patient care goals, accept and incorporate feedback, utilize scientific studies in the care of her/his patients, utilize quality improvement methods to adjust practice and participate in the education of

TABLE 3.1 A Brief Outline of the ACGME Competencies. This table was adapted from the ACGME Outcome Project.

Competency	Features
Medical Knowledge	• Knowledge about established and evolving biomedical, clinical and cognate sciences • Ability to apply this knowledge to patient care
Patient Care	• Compassionate, appropriate and effective care for the treatment of health problems • Promotion of health
Interpersonal Skills and Communication	• Effective exchange of information and collaboration with patients, families and other health professionals
Professionalism	• Commitment to ethical principles • Maintain professional responsibilities • Respectful of patient diversity
Practice-Based Learning and Improvement	• Investigation and evaluation of patients care practices • The appraisal and assimilation of scientific evidence
Systems-Based Practice	• Awareness of and responsiveness to the larger health care system • Call effectively on other resources to optimize health care

other health professionals. Competence in systems-based practice requires that learners work well within the health care delivery system, in multidisciplinary teams, in coordinating patient care and in incorporating cost awareness and risk-benefit analysis in care. The learner is also assessed on being a steward of health care resources, as well as a patient advocate.

These 6 ACGME competencies have become a standard by which residents are evaluated nationwide. They are also being used with increasing frequency to assess other medical learners, including medical students.

When I began assessing and providing remediation for struggling learners, I was at times overwhelmed by the number of deficits each individual had or by the fact that one deficit could so globally affect one's performance. I needed a framework for diagnosing learner difficulties that was concise, practical and seemed as familiar as my daily practices of diagnosing and treating patients, which is based on complaints, specifically chief complaints.

I started by exploring the framework that already existed for evaluation—these ACGME competencies. While these competencies are tremendously helpful in determining competency and levels of strength, I have broadened the list to help identify learner deficits. For example, if a learner performs poorly in the competency of patient care, it is unclear if the deficit lies in her/his clinical skills, time management and organization or clinical reasoning and judgment. For that reason, I have subdivided patient care into these 3 categories. In addition, I have separated communication and interpersonal skills. I have also added a separate competency entitled mental well-being, which includes psychosocial stressors and psychiatric diagnoses including substance abuse and learning disabilities. The expanded list of competencies will be referred to as ACGME Competencies "Plus" (see **Table 3.2**).

When considering the differential diagnosis of the struggling learner, be sure to analyze each of the ACGME Competencies "Plus," as most of our struggling learners have multiple deficits. You will find it extremely helpful to have a big picture perspective on the extent of the deficiencies. Be sure to review the entire differential and do not make any assumptions when it comes to mental health and substance use. I have heard program leadership say with confident

TABLE 3.2 Using the ACGME competencies to build a framework for the diagnosis of the struggling medical learner.

ACGME Competencies	ACGME Competencies "Plus"	
1. Medical Knowledge	1. Medical Knowledge	
2. Patient Care	2. *Clinical Skills*	Patient Care (items 2–4)
3. Interpersonal Skills and Communication	3. *Clinical Reasoning and Judgment*	
4. Professionalism	4. *Time Management and Organization*	
5. Practice-Based Learning and Improvement	5. Interpersonal Skills	
6. Systems-Based Practice	6. Communication	
	7. Professionalism	
	8. Practice-Based Learning and Improvement	
	9. Systems-Based Practice	
	10. *Mental Well-Being*	

assumption that a learner can't have a substance abuse problem because of her religious beliefs or because the learner who makes his own wine is a "true connoisseur." Don't be fooled.

You will also likely need to collect additional information to either narrow the differential or clarify the concerns. Start by interviewing the struggling learner. Ask direct questions. Systematically ask the learner about her/his skills in each competency. Treat mental well-being the same way as the other competencies to help normalize and destigmatize the topic.

Example interview of a struggling learner by a faculty member invested in remediation:

Dr. Gonzales invites Joe to meet in her brightly lit office with yellow walls peeking out around the limbs of her countless green leafy plants. Fortunately, it is a building rarely trafficked by residents, students or program faculty members, allowing for a private and confidential meeting. Joe enters, too nervous to remove his white coat, and takes a seat in the chair directly across from Dr. Gonzales. There is nothing between their chairs. A box of tissues and a pitcher of water with empty glasses sit to the side but within Joe's reach. Intentionally, Dr. Gonzales' desk is free of pen and paper, so Joe will not fear that everything he says is being written down. Notes can be taken afterward.

Dr. Gonzales: Hi Joe. Thanks for meeting with me. Let me tell you a little bit about myself. I am an internal medicine hospitalist here at the university and I work with students and residents who are either struggling or would benefit from a more individualized learning plan. Because of this role, I am here to help you and be your advocate. I will therefore not grade, evaluate or make promotion decisions regarding your education. I also help with communication between you, your evaluators and program director. I think trust is important in us being able to work together. I want you to know that I will be very transparent in letting you know what I hear and whom I speak with regarding your performance. I will be discussing general summaries of our discussion with your program director, but will not disclose any personal details.

Joe: The program director told me I had to meet with you.

Dr. Gonzales: I think I might be able to help. I'd like to start by asking you a series of questions about how you are doing on your cardiology rotation this month. I ask all learners the same set of questions, so that I don't miss anything important.

Joe: I guess it could be going better.

Dr. Gonzales: How so?

Joe: My resident and attending keep telling me that my presentations are terrible. I've been trying to improve them but I don't know how and they haven't given me any helpful suggestions.

Dr. Gonzales: What have you tried?

Joe: I've been trying to read more about my patients' diseases, but that can be difficult because my days are so long.

Dr. Gonzales: How is your medical knowledge?

Joe: I think it is pretty good. I got a 235 on USMLE Step 1 and a 222 on USMLE Step 2. (Passing >188)

Dr. Gonzales: Are you having any difficulty with performing physical exams or doing procedures?

Joe: I know how to perform the physical exam and procedures, but I have trouble deciding when they are appropriate.

Dr. Gonzales: Would you say you struggle with clinical reasoning or applying your medical knowledge?

Joe: I did really well during my third year clerkships, but then noticed there was a problem when I did my sub-internship. (i.e., a rotation in the fourth year of medical school, when a student tries to assume the responsibilities of an intern, but on a smaller number of patients.)

Dr. Gonzales: Do you have an organization system for getting through your daily tasks?

Joe: I do, but I need help creating the list and knowing what to do first.

The conversation continues, addressing time management, interpersonal skills, communication, professionalism, practice-based learning and improvement and systems-based practice individually.

Dr. Gonzales: Have you struggled in medical school other than during your sub-internship?

Joe: I did well until fourth year and ever since then I get very anxious, almost paralyzed when I have to present. I'm so worried about having to choose the pertinent information and providing a plan that I'm distracted and my mind goes blank.

Dr. Gonzales: That can be really uncomfortable. Are you feeling sad or depressed at all?

Joe: I wasn't until I was told to meet with you. I didn't realize I was performing so poorly.

Dr. Gonzales: Unfortunately, you are falling behind your peers and I want to help you before you get too far behind. Do you drink alcohol or use prescription or non-prescription medication?

Joe: Sometimes I take my wife's alprazolam and it makes me feel better, either that or I drink 2–3 beers when I get home from work. I wish I didn't have to drink at night to let down from the day.

Dr. Gonzales: Have you ever seen a therapist, psychiatrist or other doctor about your anxiety?

Joe: No.

Dr. Gonzales: Are you surprised that you are performing poorly?

Joe: No.

Notice that the faculty member did her best to create a safe learning environment, by introducing herself and her role. She also gave the learner an opportunity to speak and express his emotions freely, without fear of repercussions. Also note the use of the word "transparency" rather than "confidentiality." The idea of transparency instills trust in the process. The learners want to know who knows they are struggling and what has been said. Dr. Gonzales is not a confidential advisor and cannot promise confidentiality, as she relays general information and remediation strategies to program and course directors. She can discuss with the learner what she is going to share with others and whom she will be speaking with. This can be done without disclosing personal details, relaying only a summary of the discussion.

The learner you are trying to help might become quiet, sad, overwhelmed, angry, or defensive. Don't be surprised if the learner blames external causes or non-changeable attributes. It is important to honor his perspective and tailor your response to his emotional reaction. Some learners are very overwhelmed when they meet with me, so I spend time reassuring each of them that s/he is not alone and that I will be there to help her/him through the remediation process. Do your best to destigmatize the problem. Tell the learner how many other learners you have helped and what you have done to help them, using de-identified information. You want your demeanor to reflect that you are genuinely concerned and approachable.

If your learner gets defensive, inquire with genuine curiosity how her/his experience has not met her/his expectations. Let her/him know you are listening to what he has to say and reassure her/him that your goal and the goal of your institution is that he succeeds.

For the most resistant learners, you may have to change your tone to a more forceful one that refocuses your learner on the severity of the situation and encourages her/him to listen. In one particularly difficult encounter, I watched my mentor slap her hand firmly on the desk with earnest concern for the learner to get the learner's attention. It was extremely effective in getting her/him to listen. You have these skills. In fact, observe how you use them with patients all of the time and how these same interpersonal and communication skills can be used in working with learners who have just received bad news.

In addition to the learner, you may have to manage the emotions of those who care about the learner. I have received phone calls from lawyers, unexpected office visits from overwhelmed significant others and even emails from concerned moms. While I only give information to family members when given permission by the learner, these situations still require skillful responses and management of their emotions, as well as my own.

Lastly, you may have to support stressed, frustrated and overwhelmed faculty colleagues and program leadership. A third party objective eye, one that is not emotionally drawn into the situation, is likely to provide support and clarity as needed in developing a plan to diagnose and remediate the underperformer.

It is important to reflect on your own level of transference. Are you angry with the learner? Are your responses a result of your own frustration with the learner? Do you empathize so much that you might collude with her/his defenses? To separate your own feelings from the situation, ask yourself if your responses and actions are intended for the purpose of improving her/his performance. If not, think again about how you wish to respond or would respond differently in the future.

Let's go back to the example with Joe and Dr. Gonzales. Note that Dr. Gonzales reviews all of the diagnoses on the differential. Had she ended the interview after the clinical reasoning problem was identified, the anxiety and concerns over his substance use would have been missed. Be systematic in your interview, just like you would ask about all of the components in a thorough medical history with a patient.

If the learner provides information consistent with what you have observed and assessed or heard in reports from others, then you may breathe a sigh of relief for the process will be much easier. This learner has insight and will therefore be more helpful in creating the remediation plan and more invested in demonstrating improvement. Some learners believe that the deficiency is not theirs, blaming others or the surrounding system. Or the learner will name her/his strengths as deficits and her/his deficits as strengths. If the learner does not have insight, the remediation will require more work on self-awareness and self-motivation.

In addition to interviewing the learner, you will need to collect additional information to help analyze and narrow the differential. It may also take additional information to discover the learner's level of insight (see **Table 3.3**). As in clinical care, there is no substitute for keen observation in diagnosing your underperforming learner.

The best way to collect additional information is through *direct observation.* You can watch and assess the learner's ability to collect a history and physical and observe her/his overall efficiency, time management and organization, including her/his ability to order and prioritize tasks. Observe the learner pre-rounding in the hospital or collecting information prior to the patient encounter in clinic. This will provide a window into her/his organization and efficiency. Watch her/him after the encounter also to determine if s/he takes ownership of her/his patients and how s/he interacts with colleagues, supervisors and other members of the health care team. You may detect deficits in interpersonal skills, professionalism or even mental well-being.

TABLE 3.3 A List of Additional Resources That Can Be Used to Obtain Information About Your Struggling Learner's Performance. This information will help you narrow your differential diagnosis and identify the medical learner's specific deficit(s).

Direct Observation

- Ability to collect a history
- Ability to perform a physical exam
- Ability to collect additional patient information
- Efficiency
- Prioritizing tasks
- Responsiveness to colleagues, residents, faculty, nursing staff, etc.
- Interactions
- Ownership of patient care

Presentations/Rounds

- Integration of information
- Representation of the problem
- Formulation of DDx, assessment and plan
- Ability to summarize the case
- Formulation of questions

Interview the Learner

- Review reading materials
- Explore social stressors, mental health
- Substance abuse/use
- Learner's perspective

Other Sources

- Chart Review
- Arrival/departure time
- 360° evaluations
- Multiple choice exams
- Mini-Clinical Skills Examination
- Brief Structured Clinical Examinations
- Patient and Procedure Logs

Listening to presentations will give you a sense of whether the learner has medical knowledge, clinical reasoning skills and/or communication deficits. Can the learner integrate all of the information into a cohesive story and accurately represent the problem? Is s/he able to formulate a reasonable differential diagnosis that includes the most common illnesses and the illnesses that you wouldn't want to miss? Is s/he able to initiate a diagnostic or treatment plan? If asked to summarize a case, can s/he extract the pertinent information and communicate it in a clear and concise manner?

Aside from direct observation, consider whether additional helpful information can be gained through a chart review of the learner's patients, analysis of arrival and departure times and multi-source or 360° evaluations. The latter may provide data on her/his level of professionalism, interpersonal skills, communication, as well as time management and organization. Multiple choice exams and patient and procedure logs may also shed light on the learner's struggles.

Data collection takes additional time. If you are unable to obtain the information yourself, other faculty and chief residents can obtain this additional information with a high degree of accuracy. Having others collect information may also help maintain the learner's confidentiality in the work environment. You can ask a chief resident to round on several teams to provide feedback to the teams and at the same time collect information on the struggling learner. Or the chief can observe all of the medical students or interns to provide feedback and also collect the necessary information. If you have a well-known and recognizable faculty member who specializes in remediation, her/his presence may undermine the learner's confidentiality and trust in the program. Trust and respect for privacy are essential in making sure that the learner is treated fairly, not singled out or graded by biased faculty, and it promotes learner confidence in the system and your intentions.

Faculty at Harvard have created pre-clinical and clinical learning surveys for the learner to self-assess areas of difficulty. The learner is asked to complete the survey independently prior to initiating the interview with the remediation specialist or diagnostician. This method gives the learner time to self-reflect and participate in her/his own remediation process while helping to direct the interview and provide light on her/his level of insight. These surveys are copyrighted by the President and Fellows of Harvard College 2010, and can be obtained by contacting Laurie W. Raymond, MD at laurie_raymond@hms.harvard.edu.

While most struggling learners will have multiple deficits, it is helpful to consider how each of the individual competency deficits would present in the clinical setting (see Table 3.3).

1. Medical knowledge

Medical knowledge is the easiest deficit to identify because it can be assessed using written exams. Poor written exam scores are the most common presentation of learners with medical knowledge deficits. If you are concerned that your learner has medical knowledge deficits, but do not have access to her/his prior exam scores, ask her/him. In my experience, learners have been very honest. They often say that they have always had difficulty with exams or that they are not good test takers. If they struggle between 2 possible multiple choice answers, the learner most likely has general knowledge but lacks the specificity for the deep level of understanding that would allow her/him to use this knowledge in clinical practice.

Certainly, poor multiple choice exam scores may be from a learning disability such as dyslexia or ADHD. Asking the learner what her/his SAT scores and MCAT scores were will help you determine if this is a new problem or lifelong. This information is very valuable as it can be used when deciding on a remediation strategy. While it may be unpopular for me to say, I have yet to find a learner who has average or above average medical knowledge and poor exam scores. While the poor scores may be attributed to a learning disability, there is a good chance that the learning disability not only impacts how s/he takes exams, but also how effectively s/he is able to study.

Example of exploring a possible medical knowledge deficit:

Dr. Li: Penelope, I want to help you improve your performance. I'm trying to decide if we should spend more time working on your medical knowledge or the application of your medical knowledge. I find that exams can be a good measure of medical knowledge. Have you failed exams in the past?

Penelope: I failed my psychiatry and obstetrics/gynecology subject exams*, but passed them both the second time around.

Dr. Li: What were your United States Medical Licensing Examination (or USMLE) step 1 and 2 scores?

Penelope: I was really lucky. I passed them both the first time...by one point!

*The National Board of Medical Examiners provides subject examinations in the basic and clinical sciences for the purpose of assessing the educational achievement of individuals in specific subject areas. The subject exams are used at most LCME-accredited medical schools in the United States and Canada. Subject examinations are primarily designed for use as final examinations after courses, clerkships or other units of instruction.

Dr. Li: How did you perform on the surgery or medicine shelf exams?

Penelope: Oh, I haven't taken those yet.

Dr. Li: It sounds like we should review the medical content for this course first and then discuss application of medical knowledge.

You may also notice that these learners are unable to answer knowledge-based and fact-based questions.

Example of eliciting medical knowledge on rounds:

The attending, Dr. Li, is rounding with his ward team. The intern, John, just presented a patient with chest pain and bradycardia. Dr. Li questions the team.

Dr. Li: Which EKG leads represent the inferior portion of the heart? Penelope?

Penelope nervously looks towards her intern.

Intern John: II, III and aVF.

Dr. Li: That's correct John.

The team has moved on to the next patient, Miss Smith. Penelope has finished presenting and her leading diagnosis for Miss Smith is major depressive disorder.

Dr. Li: Okay, let's see if Miss Smith meets the criteria. Penelope, what are the diagnostic criteria for major depressive disorder?

Penelope: Hmmm...looking sad and feeling sad...like feeling more sad than she should or wants to...for too long.

Dr. Li: Tonight I want you to read the DSM IV section on major depressive disorder so that you can present the diagnostic criteria tomorrow morning on rounds.

The team has moved on to the final patient, who has a new diagnosis of Parkinson's disease.

Dr. Li: How does the typical patient with Parkinson's present to his physician?

Penelope: (whispering to the intern) Does he always ask this many questions? (announcing to the team) I'll be back. I have to use the bathroom.

You also want to see if you can detect any evidence that your learner is actively reading about her/ his patients. Trust your judgment. If it does not appear that your learner is reading then you have identified the cause of her/his medical knowledge deficit. This is a very serious and potentially career-ending condition that I refer to as "study-o-penia."

2. Clinical skills

Clinical skills deficits are most evident during direct observation. These learners leave out key physical exam elements either because they don't know how to perform them, or are unaware of the exam element or why it is important. Sometimes a weaker learner performs the exam element incorrectly or performs it correctly but obtains inaccurate information. In order to determine if the learner can differentiate rales from rhonchi or assess jugular venous pressure, you will have to observe her/him and then repeat the same exam to confirm or refute your learner's findings.

Learners who struggle with clinical skills can also have poor procedural or surgical skills. When asked specific questions, they are unable to answer technique questions about the exam or procedure. They also do not understand what information is obtained or the relevance of the information obtained from individual exam elements or procedures. They are unfamiliar with the tools of the trade and how to handle them.

Examples of clinical skills deficits:

- The learner does not know how to accurately assess and grade peripheral edema.
- The learner does not know what skin findings to look for in a patient with suspected liver disease.
- The learner does not understand the clinical significance of the chandelier sign.
- The learner does not know the anatomic landmarks for placing a subclavian triple lumen catheter.
- The learner is manually clumsy.

3. Clinical reasoning and judgment

Clinical reasoning and judgment deficits are most evident during direct observation of a patient encounter or presentation. It appears that the learner collects information and then thinks about what information has been obtained, as opposed to starting with a differential diagnosis from the beginning and refining it throughout the patient encounter. As a result, the complete history and physical is full of extraneous information while, at the same time, is missing some of the key data. This deficit is further accentuated when the learner is asked to take a focused history and complete a focused exam. These learners order too many tests because they have difficulty prioritizing the list of potential diagnoses. They struggle to rule in and rule out diagnoses based on the information collected. You may also notice that these learners rely heavily on practice algorithms, but that they cannot customize and individualize protocols and practice guidelines.

Example of a catastrophic clinical reasoning error:

Mr. Ulysses comes to the hospital with a severe, active gastrointestinal (GI) bleed and chest pain. His hemoglobin is 5g/dL. The electrocardiogram has evidence of myocardial infarction (MI) and the troponin is strongly positive. Dr. Patel, the resident with this deficit, places the following orders:

- For the GI bleed: 2 large bore IVs, IVF, type and screen, serial hematocrits, blood transfusion, nasogastric tube placement
- For the MI: serial troponins and EKGs, beta blockers, oxygen, nitroglycerin, aspirin and an IV Heparin drip with starting bolus.

If you find yourself wondering, "What the heck is she thinking?" chances are she has a clinical reasoning and judgment deficit. Of note, these students have at least adequate knowledge and good exam scores. If she does not have knowledge, then that is the primary problem rather than clinical reasoning. Her ability to clinically reason remains untested if she does not have the knowledge to exercise this skill set.

If a learner has had prior health professions training (e.g., emergency medical technician or paramedic training), he may know the next step in patient care better than her/his peers. This produces a false sense of confidence and these learners often fail to develop the necessary foundation in the basic sciences and therefore clinical reasoning to support their decisions. Eventually, the deficit becomes overwhelmingly apparent, at which point they have lost critical time in their current educational training programs required to build these skills.

In the past, educators have used models such as the SNAPPS or the the One-Minute Preceptor presentation methods to elicit and evaluate a learner's clinical reasoning and judgment skills. SNAPPS is a learner-driven method of presentation, which stands for:

S—Summarize history and findings

N—Narrow the differential to 2–3 most likely

A—Analyze the differential by comparing and contrasting

P—Plan treatment and further work-up

P—Probe the preceptor about uncertainties and alternatives

S—Select an issue related to the care for self-directed learning

This method stresses the narrowing and analysis of the differential and therefore highlights the learner's clinical reasoning and judgment. The One-Minute Preceptor is educator-driven and consists of the following: get a commitment (What do you think is going on? What do you want to do?); probe for supporting evidence; teach a general rule; reinforce what was done correctly; and correct mistakes.

4. Time management and organization

Time management and organization deficits become evident through a variety of mechanisms. These learners are often unprepared for deadlines, including the start of rounds, preparing for conferences, producing assignments, and being ready to see their subsequently scheduled patients in clinic. They are often disorganized in appearance, with pockets overflowing, spilling out pieces of paper with each step. Their presentations and written notes are missing entire sections and are out of order.

Examples of organization deficits:

- The learner's presentations and notes omit the past medical history, the family history, medications or all 3 sections.
- The learner presents the laboratory data before the physical exam or presents the vital signs with the laboratory data.

Learners who struggle with organization are often shuffling through multiple documents while presenting, trying to locate the collected information. When conveying the assessment and plan for a patient, even their thought processes are very disorganized.

Example of a struggling learner presenting the assessment and plan for a patient admitted last night:

- Markus, the student, has a deeply pensive look on his face, as if thinking intensely about the details for the first time. Markus reports, "I think the patient has acute hepatitis. Let's counsel the patient on alcohol cessation, although he does have tattoos and might have hepatitis C." Mark reaches into his pocket and pulls out even more tiny sheets of paper, 3 of which fall to the ground. He continues, "Let's check a viral hepatitis panel. And he might have fatty liver disease; hmm do I want to order an ultrasound?" Markus notices his pen is out of ink, tosses it into the basket, and reaches for another. He continues, "I'll check hepatitis B, C first, although the treatment for those is less than ideal. I had a patient with hepatitis C in my clinic and he got really depressed on treatment. I should ask this patient about mental health concerns. An alcohol level and acetaminophen level would have been helpful if I had thought about it last night." Markus smiles, confident with his performance.

If you are concerned that your learner is struggling with time management, watch what time s/he arrives in the morning and leaves at the end of the day. This can also be done through time clocks, looking to see when orders are written on patients, or when s/he uses her/his badge to enter and exit the parking garage or other restricted areas. Chances are s/he is arriving earlier and/or leaving later than her/his peers. In the clinic setting, you may notice that s/he keeps her/his patients waiting and is frequently running behind schedule. S/he may also spend patient care or otherwise dedicated time trying to get caught up on prior work.

Example of a learner who can never find enough time in the day:

- Dr. Joseph, the attending physician, has been rounding with his team on an inpatient ward service. He notices that his intern, Koichi, always looks very tired and this has gotten worse over the duration of the month. Another physician remarked that there were orders written by Koichi as late as 11PM on his non-call days. In fact one day, when Koichi had not been on call the prior night, he was noted to be wearing the same clothes, unshaved and in need of a shower. When questioned, he admitted that he had not left the prior night, as required by the new duty hours. By the time he had finished his work well after midnight, it didn't pay to drive home only to come back in again at 4AM.

5. Interpersonal skills

Interpersonal skills deficits are evident rather quickly, usually because you will hear others complaining about the underachieving learner's behavior, or that they do not like working with this particular learner. Upon observation or per report, does this learner work well with others? So much of medicine is now practiced through the interprofessional and multidisciplinary team approach that it is very apparent when a learner struggles with this competency. These learners have many more interpersonal conflicts than their peers and these conflicts are often with multiple people from a variety of roles, e.g. nurses, attendings, physician assistants, clerks and even patients. When the conflict is privately brought to the learner's attention, he almost always transfers blame to someone else. In particular, when it comes to negotiating and making compromises with staff and patients, learners with this deficit are very inflexible.

Example of interdisciplinary interpersonal skills deficit:

- The nurse, Rich, complains that whenever he pages the intern, Sue, she is rude and condescending and does not address his concerns. Upon questioning, Sue says that she is never rude and in fact it is the nurse who needs remediation. She says the nurse is always bothering her with unimportant questions or when the nurse knows that she is busy.

You may notice in this example there are also signs of deficiencies in professionalism and systems-based practice. These categories do overlap in their competency criteria. In this case, you might consider collecting additional information to determine which of the competencies is her greatest deficit.

Sometimes poor interpersonal skills are derived from past experiences, personality disorders or learning disabilities. Many very highly intelligent people who find their way into medicine have difficulty reading social cues. They do not intend to act unprofessionally and have always struggled with interpersonal interactions. Their actions and questions may seem inappropriate and their non-verbal body language incongruent, but they are earnest in their intentions. The difference between this type of learner and the unprofessional learner is that this type wants to work on her/his deficits and improve her/his ability to work and interact with others.

Because these learners struggle with working with others, they tend to adopt one of two extremes. Either they delegate and order people around, or they avoid working with others by assuming all responsibilities and expecting too little of their peers.

Lastly, specific nonproductive team interactions may be witnessed or reported to you. Does this learner yell at colleagues and staff? Do they have a reputation for blocking or "turfing" patients? Do they understand and respect personal boundaries of patients, colleagues and staff?

Example of belittling:

A senior resident, Alex, berates his intern Matt at the nurse's station for misinterpreting an electrocardiogram.

Alex: Why don't you know how to read an EKG?

Matt: Well, I usually can, but I have never seen this rhythm before. Is it AVNRT?

Alex: You either know how to read an EKG or you don't and obviously you don't. (sarcastically) Perhaps you need to repeat medical school.

When Dr. Ross pulled Alex aside to give him corrective feedback, Alex was surprised. He felt that he was teaching as he had been taught and did not realize that there were more effective ways to help his intern. Embarrassed, he promised to experiment with different teaching styles.

6. Communication

Communication deficits are often first noticed during patient presentations. These learners have knowledge, clinical reasoning and are able to organize their thoughts; however, they have extreme difficulty transmitting that information.

Their oral presentations are often poor and they are clearly not as articulate as their peers. Friendly conversations, about how the learner enjoyed her/his weekend, for example, lack fluidity. Was s/he always shy and quiet and therefore did not have a chance to develop her/his communication skills? Does s/he stutter? Does s/he use appropriate non-verbal communication, such as body language and facial expressions? Is s/he brilliant and have Asperger syndrome? Does s/he struggle to ask and answer questions? Does s/he struggle to convey compassion? Can s/he convey even basic information to her/his patients? Does s/he have to go back and see patients again or call them at home to seek information that s/he was not able to ascertain during the first encounter? Perhaps s/he has more "non-compliant" or "non-adherent" patients because s/he is difficult to understand. Is English her/his first language? If her/his presentations are missing information, s/he may not understand idioms, slang or patients with heavy accents or missing teeth. If s/he struggles to find the correct words, is s/he still thinking in her/his native language and translating into English? Is this only a verbal barrier while her/his written notes are perfectly fluent?

Example of struggles in a learner with English as a second language:

- I had known Mohamed for about a year and always thought of him as a genuinely kind young man. Then, I received feedback alleging that he did not respect women. I was surprised and requested examples. I was told that he did not consistently follow the orders given to him by women as he did with men. English was his second language, although he had almost no accent. Direct observation was invaluable. Through observation it became clear that the issue was not related to gender, but rather the form of speech. He understood direct language much more easily regardless of the gender. Males were more likely to give direct instructions, giving the appearance of a gender bias.

It is not uncommon for a learner to struggle with verbal communication, yet write perfect notes. Check the notes and charts to see if s/he is able to communicate effectively in writing. Determining whether there is a primary verbal versus generalized expressive language difficulty will help direct your remediation plan.

7. Professionalism

Professionalism deficits increase in prevalence as learners gain more experience and confidence. It, too, has several manifestations. With regard to patient care, ask yourself if this learner has poor patient-doctor relationships. Does the learner use inappropriate or condescending jargon and body language? How well does s/he know her/his patients? Look for evidence of ownership and accountability. These learners are often unable to develop longitudinal continuity with their patients or, alternatively, they develop inappropriate relationships.

Is your learner doing all of her work or taking inappropriate and dangerous shortcuts? Lazy behavior includes inappropriate timesavers as well as being late, leaving early or being absent or unreliable. As our professions adjust to shift work hours, these residents will often try to pass off inappropriate types and amounts of work to their colleagues.

Examples of unavailability:

- A nurse practitioner, Antonia, leaves the hospital 2 hours early and turns off her pager without signing out her patients or ensuring that there is someone in the hospital to cover her absence.
- A resident, Taka, does not respond to his pages in a timely manner, and avoids calling back when a patient is unstable or if it is late in the day.
- The intern, Aiden, routinely avoids returning patient phone calls at the end of clinic so that he can get to soccer practice.

Does the learner make inappropriate comments to patients, staff, colleagues or to herself? Does she make others around her uncomfortable because of her behavior? Lastly, specific unethical actions or evidence of dishonesty may be brought directly to your attention.

Examples of inappropriate behavior:

- During a patient case conference, a resident, Bjorn, asks if the patient is "a sexual deviant," referring to men who have sex with other men.
- An intern, Kraig, draws pictures of naked people and images of death and then shows his colleagues in the workroom.

- Lila, a senior resident, gets caught skiing after calling in sick and placing the work burden on another resident who has to cover.
- Sam scolds her intern in front of the attending for not calling the consult that Sam herself had agreed to call.

8. Practice-based learning and improvement

Practice-based learning and improvement deficits fall into 2 categories: the inability to accept feedback and the lack of self-directed learning. Not only do these learners not self assess their strengths and weakness, they do not seek feedback and in many cases avoid it. They either avoid private meetings with evaluators or they do not read their evaluations. If feedback is given, they are often defensive rather than genuinely eager to learn and improve. In many ways, this is the scariest scenario because the learner does not understand her/his own limitations and does not seek help when needed.

Example of a poor response to feedback:

- A faculty member, Dr. Branden, reports that a student, Joey, would get defensive when he received feedback. For example, when asked about diagnostic criteria for a disease, he answered incorrectly. When Dr. Branden made attempts to teach the correct criteria, Joey defended his incorrect answer by arguing, stating that his last teacher used different criteria.

Relating to self-directed learning, these learners do not show evidence of reading and do not look up information when questions related to patient care arise. They depend on others to give them the answers or worse...they pretend they know or they simply guess. They do not use learning goals or utilize quality improvement methods to adjust their practice.

Example of poor insight:

- In an evaluation by attending Dr. Melverson: "I am very concerned about my student, Raina. She appears to be unaware of gaps in her knowledge and instead of admitting she does not know something, she often makes up an answer. I encouraged her to conduct a quality improvement study in which she would review her own charts to help increase her awareness, but she did not think it was necessary."

9. Systems-based practice

Systems-based practice deficits can involve learning limitations related to the entire health care system. These learners struggle to function in their roles within the medical team. Sometimes they do not respect the contributions of others or they don't respect the hierarchy within the team. Learners struggling with systems-based practice often have difficulty seeking out the appropriate leader within a team, which may vary depending on the task, expertise and goal at hand. These learners often either do not know or ignore the health care resources that are available and, therefore, do not use or seek all potential health care resources for their patients. They do not consider the cost of health-care and risk benefit analyses to advocate for their patients.

Example scenario of ineffective teamwork:

The physicians, nurses, pharmacist, social worker, case manager, respiratory therapist and physical therapists gather for their daily multidisciplinary meeting. Dr. Hunter, the resident, begins:

Dr. Hunter: Okay, the first patient is Mr. Jackson in room 1201. He is here with an infection, needs a PICC line today and can go home tomorrow.

Pharmacist Dora: His "vanco" trough is 46. Can we adjust his vancomycin d....

Dr. Hunter: (interrupting Dora) Next patient, Mrs. Bloom, in 1202, is here with a pleural effusion and will need to go to a skilled nursing home. Cindy take care of that.

Social Worker Cindy: She has no insur...

The resident also fails to seek the opinion of the physical therapist. She sits quietly during the meeting, because the walker and wheelchair that she requested for the last patient were never prescribed.

Dr. Hunter: (interrupting Cindy) The last one is Mr. James in room 1207. He is being discharged this afternoon.

Dr. Hunter leaves the room.

Mr. James' Nurse Joan: ...but he just fell and broke his hip.

Example of lack of cost consciousness, being a steward of health care resources and risk-benefit analysis for patients:

- Dr. Luigi always orders antibiotics with the broadest spectrum for his patients regardless of their disease process. For example, every patient he admits to the hospital is prescribed vancomycin and piperacillin tazobactam. Upon discharge, his patients often cannot afford to fill their prescriptions, because he always chooses the most potent antibiotics and never considers cost or what the patient's insurance will cover.

Learners who struggle with systems-based practice issues may not fully understand the importance of transitions of care between practices and institutions, as well as hand-overs (aka hand-offs) between colleagues. They may leave out critical information to be shared with the patient and next provider.

10. Mental well-being

Problems with mental well-being can be the most difficult to identify. The presentation is highly variable as this category covers psychosocial stressors, psychiatry diagnoses, substance abuse and learning disabilities. If the problem is any of the first three, the biggest clue is ***inconsistent*** performance. The learner has the skills and abilities, but at times is unable to perform capably. Does s/he appear withdrawn, flat, anxious, stressed? Does the learner look different from the photo that was taken at entry into the program or school? Weight changes, fatigue, and stress may be apparent through this comparison.

Are there certain days of the week or times of the day that correlate with changes in performance? This might be a clue that the learner is using substances. When asked, does the underperforming learner endorse any of your concerns? With learning disabilities, the learner may appear to have a very isolated deficit, e.g. processing, writing, attention. Ask the learner, as they may have a history of such problems in the past and perhaps already have a diagnosis. Also, don't forget to ask about the learner's social support. This question often opens the door to valuable information about the learner's deficits.

Examples:

- Piper does not come to work and does not call to notify anyone of her absence because of profound depression.
- Bing disappears intermittently throughout the day, and twice returns with red puffy eyes.
- While the intern Maggie's performance is stellar most days, there are a few days in which she seems distracted and her performance is barely passing.
- Brayden is organized for the first 4 hours of the day and then seems scattered and has more difficulty following up on tasks.
- Sven is paralyzed at times with anxiety.

Based on a survey in the early 1990s by Patrick Hughes of 3000 residents across all specialties, 97.3% reported use of alcohol, 65.1% use of marijuana, 51.5% use of cigarettes, 29.2% cocaine, 22.7% benzodiazepines, 20.8% amphetamines, 8.2% opiates, 15.4 % psychedelics, 11.8% LSD and 8.5% barbiturates. Do not neglect to specifically address the issue of substance use and abuse. Its impact is greater than most users acknowledge. Physicians, like the rest of society, can be very ambivalent about alcohol; after all, 70% of Americans drink alcoholic beverages. A survey in 2012 among surgeons reported that those whose responses showed signs of alcoholism alone were 45% more likely to admit that they had made a major medical error in the past 3 months.

Commonly encountered learning disabilities include attention deficit hyperactivity disorder, slow reading speed and receptive and expressive language disorders. If a learner appears to have a learning disability, s/he should be formally tested so that s/he can be accurately diagnosed and treated. I will often request neuropsychiatric testing if the learner appears "unteachable" and the reason for her/his inability to learn is unclear. Testing may also be helpful after severe illness or head injury to ensure that s/he is still capable of performing the cognitive skills required of a physician. Explain to the learner that the information is needed not for the purposes of a diagnosis, but rather to improve how we teach her/him and for her/his learning and future success.

Unfortunately for the learner, neuropsychiatric testing is expensive and often not covered by health insurance. If the student or resident is unable to afford such testing, consider asking the alumni association for funding for an unexpected medical expense, requesting a scholarship or expanded financial aid. It may be financially beneficial to the institution to pay for the testing rather than lose a student or drag along a failing student or resident.

TABLE 3.4 The Presentation of Each Deficit. The chart below highlights the key notable problems associated with each aforementioned competency.

Deficit	Presentation
1. Medical Knowledge	• Unable to answer knowledge-based, fact-based questions • Lacks evidence of reading • Poor written exam scores
2. Clinical Skills	• Most evident during direct observation • Physical exams lack key elements, are performed incorrectly or inaccurate information is obtained • Does not understand what type of information is obtained by individual exam element

(continued)

TABLE 3.4 The Presentation of Each Deficit (continued)

Deficit	Presentation
2. Clinical Skills (continued)	• Poor procedural/surgical skills • Unable to answer technique questions about the exam or procedure
3. Clinical Reasoning and Judgment	• Has adequate knowledge when asked knowledge-based, fact-based questions • Good pre-clinical exam scores • Extraneous information in H&Ps • Unable to focus history and/or physical • Orders too many tests • Difficulty assigning pre- and post-test probabilities • Difficulty prioritizing the differential diagnosis and analyzing diagnoses • Difficulty individualizing protocols/practice guidelines
4. Time Management and Organization	• Unprepared • Disorganized in appearance • Disorganized presentations • Disorganized notes • Disorganized thought process • Shuffling through multiple documents on rounds • Multiple incomplete tasks • Starts earlier and/or leaves later than peers • Keeps patients waiting, frequently running behind • Spends patient care or otherwise dedicated time trying to get caught up on prior work
5. Interpersonal Skills	• Difficulty functioning within a team • High incidence of interpersonal conflicts • Frequently attempts to transfer blame • Inflexible with negotiations • Difficulty reading social cues • Awkward peer interactions • Actions and questions may seem inappropriate • May expect too much or too little from peers, nurses or ancillary support, inappropriate or lack of delegation

(continued)

TABLE 3.4 The Presentation of Each Deficit (continued)

Deficit	Presentation
5. Interpersonal Skills (continued)	• Reports of unprofessional team interactions, such as blocking/turfing patients, yelling at colleagues, or condescending or inappropriate interactions with nursing and other staff
6. Communication	• Has adequate knowledge and organizational skills • Poor oral presentations • Not as articulate as her/his peers • Struggles to answer questions, in contrast to exam scores • Struggles to convey information to patients • Difficulty formulating and asking questions • Struggles to convey variation in level of urgency and severity • Poor communication in patient charts • Needs to call patients or re-visit to obtain more information • Appears to have more "non-compliant patients" than peers (due to the learner's poor communication skills)
7. Professionalism	• Poor patient-doctor relationships • Unknown to patients • Demonstrates lack of respect • Uses technical jargon with patients • Inappropriate dress or comments • Late, absent or unreliable • Dishonest • Lazy • Specific unethical actions may be brought to your attention • Inability to develop longitudinal continuity with her/his patients • Tries to pass off inappropriate amounts of work
8. Practice-Based Learning and Improvement	• Does not show evidence of self-directed learning • Does not set personal learning and patient care goals • Does not show evidence of reading

(continued)

TABLE 3.4 The Presentation of Each Deficit (continued)

Deficit	Presentation
8. Practice-Based Learning and Improvement (continued)	• Does not utilize quality improvement methods • Not reviewing literature to answer patient care questions • Does not seek feedback • Defensive when receiving feedback • Does not understand own limitations • Does not seek help when needed
9. Systems-Based Practice	• Does not value interprofessional input • Neglects health care resources • Do not consider cost and risk-benefit analyses • Does not advocate for patients • Does not seek resources for patients • Neglects transitions of care
10. Mental Well-being	• Wide variety of problems = wide variety of presentations • Inconsistent performance

If the learner has multiple deficits, ask yourself, which ones are severe? Which ones would you consider minor? Order the list just like you would prioritize a medical differential diagnosis: the first being the most severe or the most likely to impact the learner's performance and the last being the most minor or the least likely to impact the learner's performance.

CHAPTER 4:

Diagnostic Cases

Several cases are provided in this chapter to allow you to work with these concepts and practice your new diagnostic skills. Once you are comfortable with the content, they can also be used to provide faculty development, to improve faculty's ability to observe the skills of their learners and to provide more specific feedback and accurate evaluations. If faculty development is given in the form of a workshop, have the audience play a role and read the cases aloud. Provide them with the following list of questions prior to each case.

For each case, you will be asked to answer the following:

1. Using the list below, create a differential diagnosis of the student's deficit(s) for each case and enter it into the 2nd column in the table below. List each possible diagnosis. Extend the table as necessary.
   1) Medical Knowledge
   2) Clinical Skills
   3) Clinical Reasoning and Judgment
   4) Time Management and Organization
   5) Interpersonal Skills
   6) Communication
   7) Professionalism
   8) Practice-Based Learning and Improvement
   9) Systems-Based Practice
   10) Mental Well-Being
2. Analyze your differential diagnosis (DDx). What speaks for or against each diagnosis on your differential? Fill in columns 3 and 4 in the table below. Enlarge the rows if additional space is needed.
3. What additional information or diagnostic tests would you perform to limit your differential? Add these items in the last column.
4. Consider all of the information that you have entered below. Choose ***one*** deficit to remediate. Which deficit will you attempt to remediate first?

   ____

	DDx	For	Against	Additional Info
Case #:	a.			
	b.			
	c.			

CASE 1:

In this case, a third year medical student, Wilbur, who is halfway through his family medicine clerkship, eagerly asks to present a new patient to the entire medical team. While the team has been together for 4 weeks, this is your first day attending with this learner. Just as Wilbur starts to present, the other learners roll their eyes and settle into their stances as if to prepare themselves to wait for the next blue moon. Wilbur begins enthusiastically.

Wilbur: Mr. Q is a 50-year-old Asian male who presents feeling sick. On Sunday he had a runny nose and some sneezing. Then on Monday he had a sore throat. On Tuesday he started coughing green mucous, the same type of mucous that was coming from his nose. On Wednesday he tripped on the sidewalk but didn't fall. On Thursday he started to hear whistling when he coughed. He has had colds before, just like this. Rest makes it better and smoking makes it worse.

Past Medical History

Chronic Obstructive Pulmonary Disease

Lt Ankle sprain at age 42 while playing soccer

Appendectomy at age 23, at a hospital in NYC, but he didn't know which one

Meds and Allergies

He was given a combivent inhaler 20 years ago when he went for his last physical, but he can't find it

Family History

Unknown because he was adopted

Social History

He has a 45 pack year smoking history (1.5 packs/day for 30yrs).

He smokes Camel unfiltered cigarettes.

No alcohol, no illicit drugs, unless you count marijuana

He is a postman and traveled to Italy at age 9

Physical Exam

Gen: thin male, appears older than stated age

VS: T 101°F P 105 BP 100/72 R 22 Sat 87% RA

CV: RR S1 S2 no M no edema

Lungs: Diffuse expiratory wheezing, increased A-P diameter, clubbing

EKG:

105 sinus tachycardia

CXR:

LLL infiltrate, hyperinflation and bronchial cuffing

Assessment and plan:

My differential diagnosis is: Sarcoidosis, CHF, PE, lung cancer.

All are on the differential because they cause hypoxia. Our last patient looked similar and had sarcoid. CHF and PE are common in middle aged men. Lung cancer, though maybe that should be first on the list because he is a smoker.

I think we should order:

A chest CT PE protocol
An echocardiogram and stress test
An MRI chest to look for lymphadenopathy
Consult pulmonary for bronchoscopy and biopsy
Pulmonary function tests and ABG

Let's start by giving smoking cessation, steroids, and furosemide and a heparin gtt.

QUESTIONS

1. Using the list below create a differential diagnosis of the student's deficit(s) and enter it into the 2nd column in the table below. List each possible diagnosis. Extend the table as necessary.
   1) Medical Knowledge
   2) Clinical Skills
   3) Clinical Reasoning and Judgment
   4) Time Management and Organization
   5) Interpersonal Skills
   6) Communication
   7) Professionalism
   8) Practice-Based Learning and Improvement
   9) Systems-Based Practice
   10) Mental Well-Being

2. Analyze your differential diagnosis (DDx). What speaks for or against each diagnosis on your differential? Fill in columns 3 and 4 in the table below. Enlarge the rows if additional space is needed.
3. What additional information or diagnostic tests would you perform to limit your differential? Add these items in the last column.
4. Consider all of the information that you have entered below. Choose ***one*** deficit to remediate. Which deficit will you attempt to remediate first?

____

	DDx	For	Against	Additional Info
Case 1:	a.			
	b.			
	c.			

CASE 1 REFLECTIONS:

This student's primary deficit is clinical reasoning and judgment. There is extraneous information in the H&P and the story is not represented or packaged well. Wilbur does not list the common causes of the symptoms presented, he orders too many tests and cannot prioritize what to address first. If asked, he would have difficulty assigning pre-test and post-test probabilities.

Some evaluators ask if this is a medical knowledge problem. The best way to clarify the differential would be to ask the learner fact-based questions. For example, what does COPD look like on a chest x-ray? How would you diagnose pneumonia? If the learner knows the answer, this is not a medical knowledge problem. You might also infer that the learner has sufficient medical knowledge because he knows which tests to order for each diagnosis on his differential. Though the differential diagnosis is incorrect, the learner demonstrates some knowledge.

CASE 2:

This case takes place in your outpatient office practice. This is your student's first day of her second clerkship. So far, Jane has completed her surgery clerkship. Because the patient, Mrs. Ford, is well known to you and Jane is new to both your office and the clinical family medicine rotation, you tell Jane that you want to directly observe the patient encounter. You also tell her that after she interviews Mrs. Ford, you will both leave the room to discuss the case and then return together to present the plan to the patient.

Jane knocks on the door.

Mrs. Ford: Come in

You follow the student into the room and nod to your patient, who has agreed to be seen by a student. Jane ignores Mrs. Ford, turning her back to the patient as she proceeds with washing her hands. She then sits without looking at the patient.

Jane: (rustling through the patient's chart) I hear you are feeling sad.

Mrs. Ford: Yes, my cat died 2 days ago.

Jane: I see. Have you been sleeping?

Mrs. Ford: Not very well. I often think of her at night and start to cry when I realize she is not curled up next to me.

Jane: I see. Are you still interested in activities? (Jane stiffly and nervously tries to turn towards the patient while keeping her eyes glued to the chart)

Mrs. Ford: Not really. (playing with her scarf) I used to knit, but I miss my cat wrestling with the yarn.

Jane: I see. You sound guilty. How's your energy?

Mrs. Ford: It is hard to have energy when you aren't sleeping well.

Jane: I see. How's your cognition? (Once again, trying to turn towards the patient and make eye contact)

Mrs. Ford: What does that mean?

Jane: Never mind. Do you have any psychomotor agitation? (For the first time Jane makes eye contact that lasts for less than 1 full second)

Mrs. Ford: What?

Jane: Never mind. Do you want to kill yourself or anyone else?

Mrs. Ford: No?

Jane: OK, I'm done now. (Stands up abruptly with her back towards the patient and quickly leaves the room)

QUESTIONS

1. Using the list below create a differential diagnosis of the student's deficit(s) and enter it into the 2nd column in the table below. List each possible diagnosis. Extend the table as necessary.
    1) Medical Knowledge
    2) Clinical Skills

3) Clinical Reasoning and Judgment
4) Time Management and Organization
5) Interpersonal Skills
6) Communication
7) Professionalism
8) Practice-Based Learning and Improvement
9) Systems-Based Practice
10) Mental Well-Being

2. Analyze your differential diagnosis (DDx). What speaks for or against each diagnosis on your differential? Fill in columns 3 and 4 in the table below. Enlarge the rows if additional space is needed.
3. What additional information or diagnostic tests would you perform to limit your differential? Add these items in the last column.
4. Consider all of the information that you have entered below. Choose ***one*** deficit to remediate. Which deficit will you attempt to remediate first?

____

	DDx	For	Against	Additional Info
Case 2:	a.			
	b.			
	c.			

CASE 2 REFLECTIONS:

This learner struggles with communication, interpersonal skills and perhaps mental well-being. When asked to identify the single greatest deficit, I would choose communication. Jane clearly knows what to ask and is organized in her collection of data. She senses the patient's sadness and can read her social cues, but doesn't know how to respond. Jane has difficulty choosing patient appropriate language, struggles to respond to the patient's comments and does not appear to be articulate. She also struggles with non-verbal communication, struggling with appropriate body language. Are these skills teachable? Absolutely!

Severe anxiety may also appear similar to this dialogue. Through direct observation of the encounter, it would have been clear that the student did not struggle with anxiety. You may have classified this as an interpersonal skills problem as she has difficulty relating to others. This is true. The learner, however, did not demonstrate some of the other classic features of poor interpersonal skills such as a high incidence of interpersonal conflicts, inflexibility with negotiations or difficulty reading social cues.

CASE 3:

For Case 3, there are 2 scenarios.

SCENARIO 1: In the first scenario, the setting is the oncology floor of the hospital. It captures a conversation between a resident, Dr. Lo, and the patient's nurse, Brenda.

The patient's name is Mrs. Jones and she is dying of advanced cancer. Her code status is DNAR/DNI, comfort care only, and she is scheduled to go to inpatient hospice tomorrow morning. You are Mrs. Jones' closest friend and you are at the hospital to comfort her and support Mr. Jones, the patient's husband. You and Mr. Jones were at the bedside of Mrs. Jones and witnessed her take a large gasping breath. Mrs. Jones' nurse excuses herself and leaves to page the resident.

The phone rings and the nurse answers.

Nurse Brenda: Medical oncology nurses' station. How can I help you?

Dr. Lo: It is Dr. Lo. I was paged.

Nurse Brenda: It's Brenda, Mrs. Jones' nurse. I just wanted to let you know that she just passed away. I'll grab the paperwork. Will you be able to come perform the pronouncement and talk to the family?

Dr. Lo: Yes. I'm coming.

Two minutes later, the resident, Dr. Lo, walks into the patient's room. You, Mr. Jones, and Nurse Brenda are at Mrs. Jones' bedside.

Nurse Brenda: Thank you for coming to pronounce Mrs. Jones. I told her family you were coming.

Dr. Lo: Let me see the chart. (flipping through the chart)

Mr. Jones watches the resident through his grief for any last information, hope or comfort.

Dr. Lo: (angry and yelling at Nurse Brenda) You gave her lorazepam!!!

Nurse Brenda: (matter of fact) Yes, it was ordered.

Dr. Lo: Lorazepam causes sedation and respiratory depression. Why did you give it to her? You killed the patient.

You watch Dr. Lo in disbelief.

Nurse Brenda: (shocked, there is a brief pause of disbelief, and then she replies with a timid voice)...but...you ordered it.

Dr. Lo: It was written as a PRN that means "as needed." Where was your clinical judgment? You killed her.

Nurse Brenda: This is Mr. Jones and his cousin. They have been waiting to talk to you.

Dr. Lo: I cannot believe it! (walking out of the room, not to return)

SCENARIO 2: This is the second scenario and it also occurs in the hospital, this time in the emergency room. The same resident, Dr. Lo, is present, this time with Dr. Gray, the most senior emergency room attending. Mrs. Smith was brought to the emergency room by ambulance and suffered a PEA (pulseless electrical activity) arrest in the emergency room. Cardiopulmonary resuscitation (CPR) was performed and she was resuscitated. She has a history of multiple deep venous thromboses and Antiphospholipid Antibody Syndrome. The family watches the doctors' interactions and listens in on their conversation, hoping for more information about their loved one.

Dr. Lo: Dr. Gray, I cannot believe that you think Mrs. Smith should go to the ICU.

Dr. Gray: She just had a cardiac arrest and needs monitoring for the thrombolytics that we are going to give her right now. I'm concerned that she may have a massive pulmonary embolism. I did her ECHO and her right ventricle is dilated and akinetic. I don't think the family would mind if I do the ECHO again to show you.

Dr. Lo: Lytics, that's crazy. She was dead for 10 minutes. If you give her lytics, she is just going to end up brain dead…a vegetable. That would be so much worse.

Dr. Gray: She is only 46 years old and I am fairly certain of the etiology of her arrest. Also, CPR was started immediately. She may do well. It is worth a try.

Dr. Lo: But ICU beds are limited, shouldn't we give them to someone with a better chance? And the lytics are expensive. (pointing to the family) Is the family willing to pay for them? You are just creating more suffering.

QUESTIONS

1. Using the list below create a differential diagnosis of the student's deficit(s) and enter it into the 2nd column in the table below. List each possible diagnosis. Extend the table as necessary.
   1) Medical Knowledge
   2) Clinical Skills

3) Clinical Reasoning and Judgment
4) Time Management and Organization
5) Interpersonal Skills
6) Communication
7) Professionalism
8) Practice-Based Learning and Improvement
9) Systems-Based Practice
10) Mental Well-Being

2. Analyze your differential diagnosis (DDx). What speaks for or against each diagnosis on your differential? Fill in columns 3 and 4 in the table below. Enlarge the rows if additional space is needed.
3. What additional information or diagnostic tests would you perform to limit your differential? Add these items in the last column.
4. Consider all of the information that you have entered below. Choose ***one*** deficit to remediate. Which deficit will you attempt to remediate first?

____

	DDx	For	Against	Additional Info
Case 3:	a.			
	b.			
	c.			

CASE 3 REFLECTIONS:

This case is a bit more difficult. There is clearly a problem. In fact, there may be several. To which category do we assign the deficit: interpersonal skills, professionalism and/or mental well-being? With interpersonal skills difficulties, there is a high incidence of interpersonal conflict, frequent attempts to transfer blame, deficits in reading social cues and inflexibility with negotiation. Dr. Lo had multiple high intensity conflicts with different people. When she was questioned, she blamed the other party for poor clinical judgment, did not seem to consider the option of having a private conversation and was inflexible with the range of possible treatment options and outcomes. As for her poor professionalism, the resident was disrespectful to her colleagues and didn't respect the hierarchy of medicine or the experience of the other more senior clinician. The resident was not dishonest, or lazy, nor did she arrive late or dress inappropriately.

Longitudinal information would be extremely helpful in diagnosing this learner. If the resident's performance and behaviors were erratic, or in any way inconsistent, problems related to mental well-being would have to be ruled out. This would include social stressors, psychiatric diagnoses and substance abuse. This is a case I would refer to Student Affairs, the course director, program director or remediation team for assistance with more resources to make a complete and accurate diagnosis. Resources include access to prior evaluations and clinical performance, mental health resources and substance testing if indicated.

CHAPTER 5:

Responsibilities of the Evaluator

As you are completing your student, Priya's, mid-course written evaluation, you are disheartened to realize that Priya is only 3 months away from graduation. You hear yourself whisper privately in your office, "Wow, this was the weakest student that I have ever worked with." You have identified her greatest deficit to be clinical reasoning and judgment, but what do you do next? Priya is about to move on to another rotation with another supervisor. What do you write in her evaluation? Who should you tell that you have discovered a major problem? Will it be worth your time and investment?

As an evaluator, there are many responsibilities. First and foremost, when you detect and confirm a deficiency, you must ***give the learner feedback*** as soon as possible. Let the learner know what your concerns are, with examples, and how her/his performance differs from where s/he should be at her/his level of training. Section 3 provides tips on giving effective and difficult feedback.

A learner can be assessed by comparison to her/his peers which is called norm-based assessment. Alternatively, a learner can be assessed by comparison to her/his expected level of training which is called criterion-based assessment. Norm-based assessments are very difficult for the evaluator and more likely to be biased for a variety of reasons.

- Many evaluators have not been exposed to enough learners at each level to have a true representation of the average, above average and below average learner.
- Medical teams are composed of learners from several levels and this can skew comparisons of learners (at the same level).
- Skills and abilities in each of the competencies vary by academic class, subgroups of students on clinical rotations, timing of rotations relative to overall training and by academic institution.

Criterion-based assessment is preferred because it provides constant unwavering benchmarks of performance. Criterion-based assessment tools can be used to determine if your learner is behind where s/he should be and if s/he is far enough behind to warrant the resources of intensive remediation.

If you have difficulty determining the expected level of competence, consider reviewing Lou Pangaro MD's RIME model and the non-medical Dreyfus' model. If these concepts are new to you, I would highly recommend the following articles:

Pangaro L. "A new vocabulary and other innovations for improving descriptive in-training evaluations." *Acad Med* 1999; 74(11):1203–7.

Carraccio CL. Benson BJ. Nixon LJ. Derstine PL. "From the educational bench to the clinical bedside: translating the Dreyfus developmental model to the learning of clinical skills." *Acad Med* 2008; 83(8):761–7.

Both methods are popular models for criterion-based assessment. RIME was designed in the medical education world and, while initially created for medical student education, is now being used for higher level learners. RIME stands for:

R—Reporter
I—Interpreter
M—Manager
E—Educator

Medical learners all start out as observers but when given active responsibilities, proceed along this developmental continuum. In medical education, the expectation is that medical students in their third year learn to become thorough organized collectors and reporters of information. This requires good communication and interpersonal skills, professional behavior and medical knowledge. Throughout the third year, reporters begin to transition into early interpreters. The fourth year of medical school serves to support and develop interpreter skills such as creating differentials, prioritizing and analyzing patient problems. Data now has a greater clinical significance for the interpreter. Interns and early residents manage and propose diagnostic and therapeutic options as they relate to their specific patients. The last phase is educator. Senior and chief residents and practicing physicians spend the rest of their careers improving on their abilities as educators, whether they teach in a formal academic setting, as a leader in their work environment and/or in counseling their patients.

The Dreyfus Development Model originally applied to skills such as playing chess or driving. CL Carraccio et al. wrote an article that demonstrates how these principles translate to learning clinical bedside skills. It relies on the accepted understanding of how adults learn. It is based on the notion that clinical reasoning is dependent on both an analytic (or hypothetico-deductive) approach to problem solving AND pattern-based recognition, where the ability to recognize relationships and diagnoses relies on similarities and differences to past experiences. The stages of learning in the Dreyfus Model are:

Novice
Advanced Beginner
Competent Proficient
Expert
Master

The novice level learner is rule driven, solely using the analytic reasoning approach and her/his medical knowledge to link cases and the effects. These learners have little ability to prioritize information, struggle with the volume of information that needs to be integrated and can easily miss the big picture. Each tree is fascinating, but unrelated to the larger forest. Advanced beginners sort through rules and information, using both analytic reasoning and pattern recognition. They start to abstract concepts from more concrete information. Competent learners start taking ownership of their patients and use more pattern recognition, unless a complex or uncommon patient presentation occurs. At this point, the learner would employ her/his hypothetico-deductive clinical reasoning skills. Learners at this level are able to consistently see the big picture. Proficient learners have had enough experience to feel like problem solving is intuitive. Unconsciously, they rely on prior cases using analytic reasoning as a fallback. They can easily extrapolate from a known to an unknown clinical situation. Expert and master developmental stages follow, but I will defer further explanations as these learners will likely not need remediation.

While this model is also helpful, there is not a clear consensus on which stage of education correlates with the Dreyfus stages. What stages correlate to the acquisition of individual medical clinical skills?

Let's take a look at a few cases as presented by Adam Trosterman, MD at the University of Colorado at a faculty development conference in July of 2010.

CASE 1

Emmett generates a differential diagnosis that drives the data gathering in a more focused direction. He is able to filter information and focus on the relevant data to formulate and summarize the case. He can abstract pertinent positives and negatives and appropriately incorporate them into the history of present illness. His plan seems prioritized between problems and he is able to initiate management plans, but only with the guidance of seniors on the team.

QUESTIONS

What stage of RIME is this learner? ______________________
What stage of the Dreyfus Model? ______________________
What year of medical training? ______________________

CASE 2

Melissa performs a history and physical using a set of rules. Regardless of the patient's chief complaint, she goes through each item on the generic template without gathering data on the basis of the likely differential. Each individual sign and symptom seems equally important. The pertinent positive and negative signs and symptoms are not organized but remain scattered throughout the presentation. Lastly, she links the data gathered to her knowledge from her pre-clinical studies of pathophysiology.

QUESTIONS

What stage of RIME is this learner? ______________________
What stage of the Dreyfus Model? ______________________
What year of medical training? ______________________

CASE 3

Carter can recognize patterns of illness based on previous patient encounters. He can always see the forest through the trees and the consequences of his clinical decisions. When complex or uncommon problems are encountered, he methodically attempts to reason through each step of the case, sometimes successfully and sometimes getting stuck. Carter always knows when to ask for help.

QUESTIONS

What stage of RIME is this learner? ______________________
What stage of the Dreyfus Model? ______________________
What year of medical training? ______________________

CASE ANSWERS

Case 1

RIME—Interpreter
Dreyfus—Advanced Beginner
Year of Training—4th year medical student or 2nd year of clinical medicine

Case 2

RIME—Reporter (early)

Dreyfus—Novice
Year of Training—3rd year medical student or 1st months of clinical medicine

Case 3

RIME—Manager (early)
Dreyfus—Competent
Year of Training—2nd or 3rd year resident or 4th or 5th year of clinical medicine

How do you determine the need for remediation?

Faisal is a fourth year medical student who is still an early reporter and a novice. Okay, so now I know for sure that Faisal is behind where he needs to be. But not every student can be stellar. Is he just a below average student or does he need the additional resources, in both time and money, that formal remediation will require?

Prior to reviewing the RIME and Dreyfus assessment models, the first responsibility of the evaluator is giving the learner feedback (see **Table 5.1** and Section 3). Use the provided models as a guide to determine if your learner is behind for her/his level of training and tell your learner how her/his performance compares with the established criteria for her/his level. Is s/he above in some areas and below in others? How far above or below is s/he? If you find it helpful, show her/him the assessment models so s/he can see where s/he is performing and where s/he needs to be. The visual can be very helpful for the learner to understand what you are trying to communicate and also shows her/him that you are not being arbitrary in your assessment. If s/he is one stage behind, s/he needs remediation.

TABLE 5.1 Responsibilities of the Evaluator

1. Give the learner feedback
2. Review the expectations, specific for the level of learner
3. Notify appropriate leaders
4. Provide examples
5. Do not contribute to the rumor mill
6. Document the learner's deficit(s) with examples
7. Help identify the greatest deficit and address it first

The second responsibility of the evaluator is to clarify with the learner and reiterate her/his expectations. If provided in a written or web-based document prior to the rotation, don't assume that s/he read or understood the document or that someone else spoke to her/him about it. It is always best to verbally review expectations on the first day, so that you can later refer back to what you told her/him.

Examples:

- "On the first day of this rotation when I discussed my expectations, we talked about giving at least 3 differential diagnoses for each active patient problem. You have not been doing that so it is difficult for me to give you a higher rating for 'clinical reasoning'."
- One student came to the remediation specialist complaining that her evaluation from Dr. Mensah rated her poorly because she did not see enough patients per day. Sadly, the student was never told and didn't know to ask what the expected number of patients was until the rotation was over.

Responsibility number 3 is to notify the appropriate individuals when you are concerned that a learner is behind. This is usually the course director, clerkship director or program director. For some institutions with dedicated remediation teams or remediation policies, the procedure may be different. If you are unsure of the policy, be sure to notify the director as soon as possible. It is much easier to remediate deficits early in the rotation rather than at the end of the rotation once "bad" habits have developed or, even worse, when there is limited time prior to the anticipated graduation date.

Be prepared to provide specific examples of the deficit. These are essential in convincing a learner that s/he truly has a deficit. It also allows teaching around specific events.

While it is important to notify the course leaders, tell only those who need to know. Do not contribute to the rumor mill. Let the leaders decide who else needs to know for the learner's educational benefit and patient safety. This prevents the learner from feeling targeted or isolated from his peers, and ensures that future evaluations, grades and promotions are unbiased and otherwise unaffected. It also helps promote the learner's trust in the remediation program and in the intentions of his leaders.

Most of our struggling learners have multiple deficits. In addition to identifying all of the learner's deficits try to identify the greatest. This will greatly aid the team that puts together the learner's remediation plan. This concept will be discussed more in Section 2.

Documentation of Problems...and the Pitfalls

> *It is 9PM before I even get a chance to sit down for the day. Exhausted and starving, I grab a bite to eat as I open my email. I have just received my fifth delinquency notice for not completing Nguyen's evaluation. Sarcastically, I mumble, "Great!" I wonder, should I write how I felt about working with him, what I really think about his performance or something that will subtly convey concerns without hurting his feelings? Or perhaps, I'll just fill in the rating scale and leave the comments section blank...*

How important is documentation in identifying a learner's deficits? Sixty percent of program directors felt that they had difficulty convincing residents of their deficiencies because of inadequate and/or inaccurate written evaluations. The process of reporting most often occurs via verbal comments during phone calls, private meetings or larger learner review meetings conducted by faculty and chief residents, rather than through written documentation. Although such comments are very helpful in identifying the learners in need of additional assistance and in identifying specific problems, the lack of documentation is a large pitfall.

A lack of honest and accurate written evaluations presents a unique challenge to program directors who must review evaluations as a means of monitoring their learners. The larger the program, in number of learners and sites to which they rotate, the more reliant the directors are on these evaluations in knowing how each learner is performing. Inconsistent evaluations are also challenging and represent another common pitfall. If a learner receives a high score, but the comments identify a concerning weakness, it is very difficult to convince the learner that this is a deficit that s/he really needs her/his attention.

At the University of Colorado, my colleagues and I conducted a case comparison study of the evaluations of 17 residents in good standing compared to 17 residents with a letter of warning or on probation, from 1999 to 2007. Of the residents with a letter of warning or on probation, 54.5% received evaluations with ambiguous comments, while only 18% of the residents in good standing did ($p < 0.001$). Also of note, evaluators wrote an average of 61 words in the comments for residents in poor standing versus 30 for those performing well ($p = 0.002$). When learners are struggling, it is sometimes difficult for the faculty evaluator to be direct. As a result, evaluation comments are vague and therefore ambiguous. Evaluators may write more because they are struggling to find a way to communicate their concerns. Always re-read the evaluation comments that you write. Might any of the statement be ambiguous? Ask yourself whether your comments could be perceived as either positive or negative. If you are a program director, call or e-mail the evaluator and ask her/him to clarify what s/he meant in the comments sections. Chances are, s/he will be able to tell you very clearly and bluntly what s/he was thinking.

Examples of ambiguous comments:

- "Should read more"
  - Shouldn't we all?
- "Presentation improved throughout the month"
  - Was he poor to begin with?
  - Is he now at or above the average stage of learning?
  - Was he great and got even better?
- "Better able to synthesize cases"
  - Was he unable to in the beginning?
  - Are you seeing the expected developmental improvement over an 8 week rotation?
  - Are you trying to convey that there is or was a problem?
- "Was dressed appropriately"
  - Has that been a problem with other students and you wanted to acknowledge his respect for professional appearance?
  - Were you a bit jealous of his keen fashion sense?
  - Or, was that the only positive comment you were able to offer?

We are all busy and there is never a good time to complete evaluations. But they are essential...and ***required.*** Get them in EARLY! Even though you ideally gave your learner feedback in person, many learners need the reinforcement of written comments. They also serve as documented proof if the learner denies having been told. Timeliness is essential. As a faculty member dedicated to remediation, it is heartbreaking to receive a negative comment or evaluation on a student so delayed that 3 additional rotations have gone by. Medical education is short and poor grades can be devastating to careers. The learner deserves a chance to remediate and demonstrate his successes as soon as possible, before accumulating poor scores from unknowingly repeating the same correctable mistakes.

Many evaluators are unsure of what they should document. You may document deficits on the learner's evaluations, which is preferred, or even via email to the director. Include the following:

- What are the deficiencies? (give examples)
- Where was the learner at the start and end of the rotation?

    - reference the RIME or Dreyfus stages
    - use poor, good, excellent, outstanding
    - if you must, use failing, barely passing, passing
- What do they need to continue working on?

Examples of how to document your concerns:

Example #1:

- After working with Jack for 2 weeks, I am concerned that he struggles with clinical skills. For example, while trying to place an internal jugular central line under my supervision, it became clear that he did not know the proper techniques. He was unsure how to use the neck anatomy and ultrasound to facilitate proper placement. He also struggled using the equipment in the central line placement kit. At the beginning of the 2 weeks, he was clearly below where he should be and now is barely achieving competence. I think he needs to review the technique by watching a video or reading a text and then needs to practice the procedure. I would recommend the same for placing arterial lines and chest tubes, as his technique with these procedures was also poor.

Example #2:

- Tina has shown marked improvement in her presentations. She would benefit from additional teaching on how to sort through large amounts of information. She struggles to report the pertinent questions in the history and the relevant elements of the physical exam. At times, she gets so distracted with collecting the history of present illness that she neglects to collect the laboratory and radiology data. Her RIME stage of learning is early reporter, but I expect her to be an interpreter at this stage. She is making progress, but would benefit from continued work in this area.

Note that the first sentence in example #2 is very ambiguous, in terms of determining whether she is in need of remediation. Fortunately, the remainder of the paragraph is clarifying and very specific.

Example #3:

- Jennifer seems to struggle with communication, both with patients and on rounds. Due to my limited time attending on this rotation and our limited interactions, it is difficult for me to assess her completely. I am concerned that her skills are not that of a fourth year medical student and that she may need further assessment in this area.

As highlighted in example #3, you do not need to have all of the answers. It is acceptable to qualify your concerns if you are unsure. Most importantly, you have brought your concerns to the attention of the individual reviewing and compiling evaluative information.

Lastly, let your evaluators know how the institution responds to the negative or corrective comments that they write. They are more likely to write comments if they know that they will truly be used to help the learner succeed. Do your best to avoid the common pitfalls (see **Table 5.2**).

Program, clerkship and course directors who are not getting what they need from faculty need to build a new culture and teach them. Evaluators need to be educated to help overcome the pitfalls and provide the type of information that would be most helpful. A description of the remediation program at my institution is readily available to graders and educators. Much of the information in this text has been provided in the form of grand rounds and is regularly dispersed at faculty development workshops on our campus and at professional society meetings. Not only has it helped to build the program, it has shifted the culture, including faculty's and administrators' views on remediation. It has

TABLE 5.2 Common Avoidable Evaluation Pitfalls

1. Learners determined to have some deficiency requiring remediation receive no post-rotation performance rating
2. Learners determined to have some deficiency requiring remediation receive no post-rotation performance evaluation indicating that deficiency
3. Written comments on the evaluations are not consistent with the numeric rating scale (Written comments are more likely to detect a deficit)
4. Evaluators lack the willingness to record negative evaluations
5. Evaluations are delayed or too infrequent to assess the problems
6. Evaluators don't know what to write when a student is struggling
7. Evaluators want to know that there is a plan in place before they document poor evaluations
8. Evaluators use inappropriate or ineffective communication methods that circumvent direct feedback to the learner (e.g., email to program director rather than comment on evaluation form)

helped educate teachers on what to look for in their learners and has ensured that the faculty know whom to contact and from whom to ask for help early on.

Identification is the key. It is both professionally and ethically essential that deficiencies are directly and clearly communicated to the learners having difficulty and to program leadership. The learners deserve timely and honest constructive identification of problems to allow them to demonstrate mastery of the solution, to avoid recurrences, ensure patient safety, and prevent professional liability. The program leadership deserves to have accurate assessments of their learners for remediation, curriculum design, and for creating a vision and building the direction of the program.

KNOW the Warning Signs

If, during the identification and diagnostic process, you notice any of the issues below, you must seek higher level help *immediately*. This may be the course leader, program director or appropriate deans. Be prepared to contact any of these individuals using their cell phones, home phones, pagers or texts (even if it is a holiday weekend). Be sure that your page or text was received. Circumstances warranting immediate intervention include:

- The learner cannot continue caring for patients safely
- The learner is not capable of learning given the circumstances
- The learner is a danger to herself/himself or others
- The learner is greatly impeding the learning environment for other residents and students
- The learner cannot continue to teach her/his peers and students, if that is part of her/his role

Self-Assessment Quiz for Section 1

It is your second day attending on the internal medicine inpatient ward service. The residents and students have been working together for the past 2 weeks. You arrive on the general medical floor of the hospital at 9AM, wait for the team for 5 minutes and then decide to begin rounds.

Attending: It is 5 minutes after 9. I know everyone is not here, but let's start rounds...

Student, Kris, comes running up from the back of the room, pockets overflowing, collar partly tucked in.

Attending: You're late, again. Rounds start at 9 o'clock.

Kris: Sorry… but I remembered my white coat today (smiling sheepishly).

Attending: You are up first. Please present Mr. Mathes.

Kris: Okay. (taking a deep breath) A 50-year-old male presents with a cough. One week ago, he developed rhinorrhea, sneezing, and a sore throat. On the 3rd or 4th day the cough started. It is productive of green sputum and wheezing. The wheezing is like when he has his asthma attacks. Well, he calls it asthma, but the medical record says chronic obstructive pulmonary disease. And he says he has a fever, but his temperature here was only 97°F. Or do you prefer Celsius? Smoking makes his symptoms worse. You know he has been smoking since he was 9 years old, unfiltered cigarettes. And you can tell when you hear the rhonchi and wheezing in his lungs. Surprisingly though it is hard to localize the pneumonia that showed up on his chest x-ray.

Meds and Allergies

He was given a combivent inhaler 20 years ago when he went for his last physical, but he can't find it. I know what that's like

FmHx

Unknown as he was adopted

SocHx

45 pack year smoking history (1.5 packs/day for 30 years)

No alcohol, no illicit drugs, unless you count marijuana

He was recently discharged from prison and that makes me think he has TB or maybe an HIV-related pneumonia

Physical Exam

Gen: thin male, appears older than stated age

Lungs: Diffuse expiratory wheezing, rhonchi increased A-P diameter, clubbing

CXR:

LLL infiltrate, hyperinflation and bronchial cuffing

CV: RR S1 S2 no M no edema_

EKG:

105 sinus tachycardia

Assessment and plan:

The differential diagnosis included pneumonia, bronchitis, and upper respiratory infection

Oh, and his white count is 15, with a left shift

Let's start Ceftriaxone and Azithromycin
Or maybe the infiltrate is cancer. Let's get a CT scan
Then he would only need inhalers for now
But he is febrile, so let's restart the antibiotics with the inhalers
Did I tell you he is HIV positive?...I think I may have left that out

Before beginning the questions, remember back to case 1 from chapter 4. Notice that there are some similarities and some differences in the presentation of the same exact patient.

1. Does Kris have a deficit?
   a. Likely
   b. Probably Not
2. Assuming that this is representative of his prior performance; do you have a framework for diagnosing the deficiency?
   a. Yes
   b. No
3. You are a skilled clinician who routinely creates differential diagnoses for your patients' problems. Create a differential for this learner's deficit(s). Circle all that apply:
   1. Medical Knowledge
   2. Clinical Skills
   3. Clinical Reasoning and Judgment
   4. Time Management and Organization
   5. Interpersonal Skills
   6. Communication
   7. Professionalism
   8. Practice-Based Learning and Improvement
   9. Systems-Based Practice
   10. Mental Well Being
4. In the real world, you could collect more data to narrow your differential. Based on the scenario, what deficiency should the remediation target?
   a. Clinical Skills
   b. Practice-Based Learning and Improvement
   c. Time Management and Organization
   d. Time Management and Organization and Professionalism

e. Professionalism and Mental Well-being
f. Time Management and Organization and Mental Well-being

5. For this case, you want to communicate your diagnosis of the learner's deficiency. Choose the BEST answer.
   a. You should notify the course director as soon as possible via email with the deficits, greatest deficit and examples
   b. You should discuss the learner's performance with the course director at the next meeting that you both attend
   c. You should notify the course director through the end of clerkship evaluation with the deficits, greatest deficit and examples
6. As the evaluator, you must notify the program leadership at home on a Saturday night via cell phone if: (check all that apply)
   a. The learner cannot continue caring for patients safely
   b. The learner is not capable of learning given the circumstances
   c. The learner is a danger to him or herself or others
   d. The learner is greatly impeding the learning environment for other residents and students
   e. The other learners on the team don't want to work with this learner

Section 1 Self-Assessment Answers

1. (a) Likely
2. (a) Yes, use ACGME Competencies "Plus"
3. (4), (7), (10) Although there may be additional reasonable answers, the top 3 include: Time Management and Organization, Professionalism, Mental Well-being
4. (c) The take home message is to choose one competency to remediate at a time.
5. (a) Early notification with documentation is crucial.
6. (a) and (c) If patient safety is a concern, do not wait until Monday even if you give the learner Sunday off, as that does not guarantee that the learner would not be involved in patient care. Troubled learners sometimes show up anyway, or make their way onto other services. If learner safety is an issue, or the safety of others, time is of the essence.

SECTION 2:

Remediation of the Struggling Medical Learner

Defeat is not the worst of failures.
Not to have tried is the true failure.

George Edward Woodberry*

*From Cane, Melville. "George Edward Woodberry: A Student's Memories." *Prairie Schooner* 1948 (22.3): 292–298.

CHAPTER 6:

Introduction and Initial Steps to Remediation

You have suspected that Ty's performance was less than stellar, but you have not had any definitive evidence or evaluations until now. You are frustrated by the delay in identification and you are eager to begin remediation with him as soon as possible. You page Ty to your office and open up your favorite remediation guide to choose a remediation strategy.

If you have jumped ahead to this section, you have been caught! It is strongly recommended that you read through Section 1 prior to reading about the remediation of the struggling medical learner; otherwise, you may not have the proper framework to proceed.

Now that you have read the first section, please take a moment to reflect on how remediation is different from traditional teaching.

____

____

____

____

____

____

____

____

Teaching involves imparting new knowledge and skills to your learner, while remediation focuses on the correction of skills. Remediation implies that there is a need to remedy errors, by clarifying what was learned incorrectly or was not learned the first time around. Those who need remediation have fallen behind their peers, either through failure to improve or by improving at a slower rate than sufficient to keep up with the curriculum. Remediation tends to be more individualized and focused on isolated deficits. It requires additional resources and is often time pressured and relies more heavily on learner insight than does teaching.

This section is written to aid individual teachers, including faculty and chief residents and course and program leaders. While some information applies more to a subset of faculty dedicated to remediation, the vast majority of information will be useful to all parties. I would encourage all faculty members to at least initiate remediation when there is a deficit, even if a formal process isn't in place yet. Please know that remediation can begin before any formal meeting has been convened, or before a remediation plan has been finalized.

To formalize the process, there is a step-by-step approach that can be used when learner concerns are brought to your attention. Faculty can use it when a resident, fellow learner or nurse tells you about a struggling learner. A course director or program director can also use it when a faculty member voices concerns about a learner.

Step 1: Request documentation and examples

Step 2: Notify and discuss the learner's performance with ONLY those who need to know

Step 3: Confirm the concerns and collect more information as needed

Step 4: Decide

- Is this a trend that needs intervention?
- Is this an isolated serious problem that needs intervention?
- Does this concern warrant only monitoring at this point?

Step 5: Make sure the learner receives direct feedback of the deficit(s)

- Often, you may have to do this yourself
- Examples of poor performance are essential, especially if you were not present when the deficit was noticed

---

Example 1:

The clerkship director, Dr. Smart, is working at her desk, when a resident appears in the doorway. Dan, the resident, looks anxious and tentative. It is unlike him to just show up at the clerkship director's office unannounced.

Dan: Hi Dr. Smart!

Dr. Smart: Hello. Come on in and have a seat. How can I help you?

The resident enters her office, closes the door behind him and takes a seat.

Dan: I'm concerned about the medical student on my team this month.

Dr. Smart: How so?

Dan: Her medical knowledge is weak.

Dr. Smart: Can you give me an example?

Dan: She doesn't know the differences between asthma and COPD. She can't explain the physiology, common presentations, or features of either diagnosis.

Dr. Smart: Is it just pulmonary diseases?

Dan: No, renal failure and liver disease are worse. She does know a lot about heart disease, as she wants to be a cardiologist and has done research on rat hearts.

Dr. Smart: If you don't mind, I would like to talk to your attending and ask him how everyone on the team is doing. I suspect he will identify the same concerns.

Dan: All right.

Dr. Smart: I also want to talk with the student. So as to maintain your confidentiality, I will tell her that the team is concerned with her knowledge and I will inquire how she has done in her prior blocks and courses. I also want to make sure that she knows what to be studying for this rotation.

Dan: Thank you.

Dr. Smart: Thank you. Oh, and would you mind sending me a brief email with your current concerns now and a follow up email in 2 weeks to let me know how you think she is doing?

Dan: I can do that.

Example 2:

The program director is precepting residents in clinic. A concerned resident, Tibor, who is mature and well respected in the residency program for being a leader and future chief, approaches her.

Tibor: Hi Dr. Chenouda.

Dr. Chenouda: Hi. How is third year treating you?

Tibor: Good...do you mind if we find a private place to talk?

Dr. Chenouda: Not a problem. Let's go into Doug's office. He is not here this afternoon.

They enter Doug's office, close the door and have a seat.

Dr. Chenouda: Is everything okay?

Tibor: (in lightning fast speed) Yes...but I'm concerned about one of the interns on my team this month. I'm currently rotating at St. Patrick's hospital on the cardiology service.

Dr. Chenouda: How so?

Tibor: Her presentations are so disorganized and she is really anxious.

Dr. Chenouda: Can you give me an example?

Tibor: Sonja definitely understands what is going on with her patients, but every piece of her presentation comes with a bit of commentary related to the suspected diagnosis or plan. The information just seems to be in the wrong sections.

Dr. Chenouda: Is her problem with organization limited to her presentations?

Tibor: No, I have to help her keep track of her daily tasks as well. I taught her my check-box system for organization and I think that it is helping her get things done and to not be so overwhelmed.

Dr. Chenouda: If you don't mind, I would like to talk to your attending and ask him how everyone on the team is doing. I suspect he will identify the same concerns. I will also ask the chief resident to round with each of the post-call teams this week, so that we can come up with a plan to help her. Would that be okay?

Tibor: Yes, thank you.

Dr. Chenouda: Thank you. Oh, and would you mind sending me a brief email with your current concerns now and a follow up email in 2 weeks to let me know how you think Sonja is doing?

Tibor: Sure, I will do that.

Notice how intentionally Drs. Smart and Chenouda describe or demonstrate how they are going to preserve the reporter's confidentiality and the learner's privacy. They are trying to protect the reporter from negative repercussions and create a safe environment for reporters in training. Also, they are trying to prevent the Pygmalion or Rosenthal effect. In the historic Oak School experiment, teachers were led to believe that certain elementary school students were more likely to demonstrate higher rates of intellectual growth and development. These students, however, were selected at random and not based on any perceived potential. The students with the higher expectations showed significantly greater gains in intellectual growth than did those in the control group. J Rheum wrote, "Simply put, when teachers expect students to do well and show intellectual growth, they do; when teachers do not have such expectations, performance and growth are not so encouraged and may in fact be discouraged in a variety of ways." Hence, the remediation program should strive to limit the number of people who are aware of the learner's need for remediation. During the remediation process and development of the remediation plan, I encourage and empower the learner to let the team and faculty know what they want to work on for the week or rotation. The learner refers to her/his remediation needs as her/his education goals, which does not identify them as in remediation but does help her/him get the focused attention where s/he needs it.

These 2 examples address Steps 1 through 3 above. Steps 4 and 5 can be addressed after more information has been collected.

Example 2 continues...

Dr. Chenouda calls the chief resident, Vimala, to observe each team round and to give her feedback on the teams. One week later Vimala meets with Dr. Chenouda.

Vimala: Hi Dr. Chenouda. The teams were interesting to watch, as they all function so differently. I did notice that one of the interns, Sonja, is struggling a bit with organization. I talked to my co-chief Martin, and he said she struggled with the same thing last month when she was on her intensive care unit rotation at the University Hospital, but he and her attending thought it had to do with the volume of data specific to that unit.

Dr. Chenouda: Can you give me an example from your observations?

Vimala: Sonja's presentations were completely out of order, and she told me that she was violating work hours to complete her tasks almost every day. And, yes, I gave her very specific feedback about my concerns. I told her...

Now you can move to Steps 4 and 5. Sonja's difficulties are serious in that they have persisted longitudinally in various environments and are impacting her ability to maintain work-life balance. Fortunately, Vimala gave Sonja feedback, which you can reinforce at your meeting with Sonja. Just because Vimala gave Sonja feedback, it doesn't mean that Sonja heard it. Talk to Sonja about the feedback she has received, and then specifically mention Vimala's feedback to ensure that she remembers having heard it. If not, this is your chance to reiterate what was conveyed and to send Sonja a follow-up email regarding your discussion.

CHAPTER 7:
Goals of Remediation

For the first time ever, I was asked to remediate a student who had genuinely failed all of the competencies, including mental well-being. Despite having worked with over 160 struggling learners, I came home completely overwhelmed. I told my wife, "I just reviewed the record and evaluations of a learner who has deficits in every possible category. Where do I start?" Clearly, she has been listening for years. She said, "Start with the ONE greatest deficit."

The goal of remediation is to target and fix the greatest deficit. Most learners have multiple areas of deficiency. Do not get overwhelmed even by learners who have deficiencies in all 10 of the ACGME Competencies "Plus". Try your best to stay calm. Just follow the rule that I learned from Jeff Wiese, MD: Choose the one deficit that you believe will yield the greatest return for the efforts invested. **The goal of remediation is to target and fix the greatest deficit.**

Choosing one category gives the teacher and the learner a defined problem to address and a place to concentrate all remediation efforts. Tackling one deficit at a time is less overwhelming for the learner and is more likely to yield success. With each incremental improvement, the learner gains confidence and the process is positively reinforced. Once one deficit is improved, momentum continues to help improve other areas of deficiency, one at a time. Targeting one problem also allows the learner to focus her/his attention on one problem and demonstrate mastery in that area. This will improve the learner's overall performance, confidence and motivation to improve, which will lead to the correction of other deficits.

Say, for example, a resident is struggling with both clinical reasoning and time management. His inability to make clinical decisions is slowing him down and making him more inefficient. Fixing clinical reasoning lends itself to remediating his time management skills next.

There are a few caveats to choosing the greatest deficit to address first. If mental well-being or professionalism deficits are noted, consider starting there. There's no sense in working on another area if the learner is in a state that won't allow her/him to be taught. If the learner just doesn't have enough medical knowledge to engage in clinical reasoning, then start with the remediation of medical knowledge. Sometimes you need to work with the learner's willingness to participate and, in this case, you may let the learner choose where to begin.

While it is very important to decide which of the learner's deficits is the greatest, do not over think it! If you choose the "wrong" place to start, you will either make progress regardless or you will quickly realize and redirect your remediation strategies.

Who should be involved in developing a remediation plan?

All formal remediation plans should be developed through a team approach. For each learner requiring remediation, a "Success Team" is convened for a meeting that may include the course or program director, faculty member(s) who have worked closely with the learner, a remediation team or faculty member specializing in remediation and, most importantly, the learner in difficulty. Unless your program is very small, the members of the "Success Team" should not be in the position of grading or promoting the learner, as this could represent a conflict of interest. It could impact the learner's willingness to be totally upfront in the remediation process, impact the creation of a safe learning environment for a potentially tentative learner and impact the subsequent assignment of grades.

While a team is tremendously helpful for the most challenged learners, this does not mean a teacher or a learner cannot use these strategies outside a formalized team approach.

As an active participant in the remediation process, the learner will be required to complete a verbal or written self-assessment regarding her/his performance. Her/his self-assessment is then discussed with either the entire "Success Team" or with a member of this team. This self-assessment should include suggestions from the learner on her/his strengths and weaknesses and how s/he can improve upon her/his deficits. Involving the learner in the remediation process will allow the program to determine the learner's level of insight into her/his difficulties and her/his willingness to participate. It will also allow the learner to have some control over the future of her/his career and provides an additional perspective as to which modes of remediation may be most helpful.

Historically, based on a literature review and discussions with a variety of programmatic leadership, remediation interventions have included a variety of the following interventions:

- Program director/Clerkship director/Course leader
  - Facilitate an advisor/advisee system
  - Make schedule changes to reduce stress and/or ease time demands
  - Make schedule changes to support the learning needs of the learner
  - Schedule repeat rotations/extending training
  - Issue letter of warning/focused review[1] or probation
- Supervising Attending
  - Provide orientation and communication of expectations at the beginning of each rotation
  - Give prompt specific feedback and discussion of concerns
  - Serve as a role model
  - Enforce behavior guidelines
- Faculty Mentor for Remediation
  - Provide core content review with tests or specific skills training
  - Review charts with learner
  - Recommend behavior guidelines
  - Conduct videotaped encounters and provide the learner with feedback
- Mental Health Service
  - Promote self-awareness and care
  - Federation of State Physician Health Programs (FSPHP.org)
    - Addressing secondary causes of poor performance (the D's): Learning disability, Depression, Distraction, Deprivation, Drugs, Disorder of personality (personality disorder)
    - Offer stress management classes
    - Formal rehabilitation of substance abuse
    - Arrange support groups for residents, though this may affect anonymity

Frequent, accurate and direct feedback and working with a mentor are thought to be the most helpful interventions. In Saxena, et al.'s study entitled "Remediation Techniques for Student Performance Problems After a Comprehensive Clinical Skills Assessment," precepted video review was most frequently used and clinical activities were the least used. Confidence in the effectiveness of the school's remediation process was significant and positively

[1]"Focused Review" is essentially the same as a letter of warning. Licensing agents, credentialing committees and review boards have become savvier and now often ask not only about prior probationary status but also about any prior warnings. Many programs no longer use the word warning so as to keep the concern internal.

correlated with the overall effort toward remediation. There was highest confidence in using standardized patients, workshops, seminars and group discussion for the remediation of deficits. It is unclear how much confidence correlates with effectiveness, providing a ripe area for research.

The experience and expertise of the author and review of the existing literature led to the development of deficit-specific remediation algorithms, which have been used successfully at the University of Colorado for the remediation of over 160 medical learners across the continuum of medical education levels from student through practicing clinicians. The use of outcomes data to support this method is discussed in the last chapter.

CHAPTER 8:

Deficit-Specific Remediation Algorithms

Please notice as you read and work through each of these approaches that there are 3 universal components as recommended by Karen E. Hauer, MD: deliberate practice; feedback; self-assessment (see **Table 8.1**).

TABLE 8.1 Three Key Principles for Building a Remediation Plan

1. Deliberate Practice
2. Feedback
3. Self-Assessment

Deliberate practice is a distinct concept that has been researched and further developed by K. Anders Ericsson. If you have read the book *Outliers* by Malcolm Gladwell, then you will see how his "10,000 hour rule" relates to the concept of deliberate practice. Deliberate practice involves performing a skill repetitively, each time receiving and incorporating external and internal feedback to improve one's ability to master that skill. This requires one to use the feedback and self-assessment to create a new action plan for improving his practice of that skill.

Deliberate practice of the weakest skill improves this deficit by gaining more experience and exposure. Because learners of all abilities are notoriously poor self-evaluators, they need to receive specific reinforcing and corrective feedback. The term feedback is meant to include demonstrating, advising, critiquing and questioning. Lastly, learners need to reflect on their performance. What works? What doesn't work? How does one's behavior/practice differ from her/his colleagues or more senior role models? Such reflective dialogue with a mentor helps the learner see other perspectives and approaches, and consider alternative strategies.

All 3 are necessary because human behavior is mediated by what people know and think. Knowledge is necessary but not sufficient to cause a change in behavior; and behavior is influenced by individual beliefs, motivations, skill and environment.

A step-by-step approach is outlined for each of the deficits in the ACGME Competencies "Plus," as described in Chapter 3. Some of the algorithms involve many steps. After each meeting with the struggling learner, you will want to send an email to document your discussion in general terms, what steps you have covered, the educational pearls provided, the learner's responsibilities prior to the next meeting and the date of the next meeting. I cannot emphasize enough the value of these emails as they promote clear communication of expectations, orient the learner to her/his role and stage within the remediation plan and provide legal documentation of all efforts.

Additional measures for promoting success include providing the learner in remediation with a supportive environment (see **Table 8.2**). The learner needs to know that s/he has permission to change and that there is an expectation that s/he can and will improve and grow personally and professionally. In order to succeed, the learner will need challenges that are of reasonable size and difficulty. Being called in for remediation is jarring to one's confidence, ego and self-image. S/he needs to feel the support of her/his faculty and peers as s/he rides the roller coaster of emotions associated with remediation, the most common of which is depression. There is also a sense of loss of control, so whenever possible allow your learner to have some choice and let them assume responsibility for her/his future.

Lastly, you may find it extremely helpful to identify the methods that are most effective for teaching your learner. You can start by asking: how do you learn best, i.e. what study methods have worked successfully for you in the past? Some learners are visual learners, others auditory and other are hands-on learners. Some learners need to understand the details and mechanisms to understand the big picture, others need the big picture framework to understand the smaller details. Or you can take a more structured approach as there are 4 dimensions of learning preferences:

1) sensing (concrete) or intuitive (abstract)
2) visual (seeing) or verbal (hearing)
3) active or reflective
4) sequential (left brain) or global (right brain)

TABLE 8.2 Ways to Promote Success in your Learners

1. Permission to Change
2. Expectation of Growth
3. Reasonable Challenges
4. Connection to Faculty and Peers
5. Choice

You or the tutoring remediation specialist may find it helpful to determine your learner's preferred learning style. Consider using either the 44 item Index of Learning Styles (ILS) questionnaire (available on the Web for free at www.engr.ncsu.edu/learningstyles/ilsweb.html) or the VARK (Verbal, Aural, Read/Write, Kinesthetic) inventory (available at www.vark-learn.com). The remediation algorithm you choose can then be tailored to increase the effectiveness for your individual learner.

1. Step-by-Step Approach to the Remediation of Medical Knowledge

Medical knowledge, including poor standardized exam scores, is one of the easiest competencies to remediate as long as you have an invested learner (see **Table 8.4** on page 100). It requires relatively minimal financial costs and faculty time. There are also many resources available, depending on the knowledge deficit, to aid the learner. It does, however, require commitment and discipline on the part of the learner, and for the learner to be held to task such as with a study schedule or periodic exams. It may also require you to troubleshoot overcoming prior barriers to studying and, as previously mentioned, determine the method by which your learner learns best.

1. Meet with the Success Team to review the remediation plan, methods for learner reassessment and goals for successful remediation
   a. Program, clerkship or course director
   b. Faculty interested in leading the remediation
   c. The learner
2. Identify knowledge gaps
   a. Review learner performance on prior standardized tests (SAT, MCAT, USMLEs) and written course exams
      i. If the student has done well in the past
         1. chances are s/he has the necessary skills and likely just needs to put in more time reading and studying
         2. or, there was a traumatic event that changed her/his ability to perform like a head injury, physical illness or treatment (meningitis, chemotherapy) or mental illness (depression or anxiety) that s/he will be able to identify for you
      ii. If the student has always struggled, s/he will need a new study method
   b. Ask the learner to identify knowledge gaps
   c. Is this problem global or specific to a topic?

   d. You may need to further test the learner through written exams to determine depth and breadth of knowledge deficits or to identify specific needs
3. Compare the learner's knowledge gaps with the course requirements and identify where they overlap
4. Establish and communicate to the learner how they will be reassessed and what is required to pass the course
   a. Where possible, establish an objective and specific score or percentile on an in-service exam, shelf exam, department exam or published question banks
   b. Be sure to include the required passing score up front
5. Review what the student is reading
   a. Recommend review material rather than primary articles
   b. Assess whether the learner has chosen the appropriate amount of material to cover, neither too little nor too much
   c. Change from disease-based reading to symptom-based reading
      i. For example, have the student read about the approach to a patient with shortness of breath rather than reading about pneumonia
   d. Let the learner know how many times s/he should review the material or how many practice questions s/he should complete prior to an exam or completion of a course
6. Identify medical knowledge goals for a given time frame and set up a study schedule with the learner
   a. What material should be previewed prior to, during and after the educational experience?
      i. Try to align the study schedule with course content or specific clinical rotations for reinforcement, such as reading about renal while on his renal elective and cardiology while on his cardiac intensive care rotation
   b. If the schedule spans months or years, consider including break time to give your learner a break or a chance to catch up if s/he falls behind with his studying
7. Encourage active learning
   a. If the learner prefers visual teaching to reading, such resources are available. Also have the learner create his own visual maps, charts, pictures and algorithms from the content they extract from their reading
   b. If the learner is an auditory learner, s/he will likely prefer discussion. Help the learner set up or find a study group. S/he can also audio record herself/himself dictating what s/he just learned, and then listen to her/his own recording over and over

c. If the learner prefers to read, encourage her/him to keep a written (not typed) record of the things that s/he does not know. Once s/he has gotten through the material for your course, s/he can review her/his written record and continue to distill it down to smaller records of what s/he still can't remember. Usually 3 distillations are necessary. This will prevent her/him from returning to the main source text and spending time on content that s/he already knows

8. Emphasize the importance of understanding
   a. Direct the learner to understand why and when, rather than how or what to do next
   b. Emphasize learning over knowing
   c. Encourage the learner to compare and contrast diseases with similar presentations
      i. For example, why do patients with chronic obstructive pulmonary disease (COPD) gradually become hypoxic throughout their lives and patients with asthma typically do not? Or why do patients with COPD have elevated bicarbs on their chemistries and patients with asthma do not?
9. Encourage the learner to link reading to patient cases
   a. Bring that material to discussions, rounds, and presentations to further solidify concepts
10. In the clinical setting, encourage self-reflection by having the learner create an ongoing list of questions that require answers
    a. Require that this homework be done at the end of each day, either memorizing facts and/or looking up facts
    b. You may need to help the learner identify learning topics
11. Remediation in the form of tutoring for specific knowledge content deficits may be necessary, especially if the learner can memorize but not understand concepts or is an auditory learner
12. Have the student reflect on her/his progress and give feedback regularly
    a. Include monitoring to make sure the student is following the recommended approach and study schedule
13. Encourage the learner to limit caffeine and other over the counter medications, and get *at least* 6 hours of sleep per night.
    a. You may need to recommend medical evaluation or psychiatric evaluation for sleep problems

14 Help the learner identify her/his most productive time of day for studying

15. Accommodations may be necessary if the student has a disability or is too far behind to get caught up within your course timeframe

16. For difficulties with exams
    a. If the learner is unable to complete exams in time, the problem may be that s/he has a slow reading rate. S/he will need to do many more practice questions than her/his peers
    b. If s/he gets distracted while reading a question, have her/him read the last line of the question block to know what the question is asking and then go back and read the body of the question
    c. If s/he is consistently able to narrow the answer down to 2 choices, but has difficulty choosing the correct answer, then s/he lacks specificity in her/his knowledge and needs to spend more time with the details after s/he understand the big picture
17. Consider further assessment from a learning specialist or neuropsychiatric testing if the learner appears to be "unteachable" despite her/his earnest efforts

---

Example:

Upon the request of the division head, I met with an attending physician, Dr. Kiersten, who was perplexed as to why she had failed her specialty boards multiple times. In this case, only Dr. Kiersten and I, as the remediation specialist, met to develop a remediation plan. I asked her to bring her test results from the prior exams which showed very low scores in all but 2 categories. The areas in which she had scored well were areas in which she had either done research or had more clinical training. Since she was able to excel in 2 areas, I thought perhaps general test taking wasn't the problem but rather content knowledge in the other areas. I also asked her about prior standardized exam performances, all of which she had barely passed.

I asked Dr. Kiersten what she had done to study for the exam and she reported that she had two different well-known review book series and ample practice questions. So I asked, "How much of the material did you review prior to the exam?" She replied, "I read some of each chapter and completed 175 questions." Shocked and thinking that perhaps I had heard her incorrectly, I repeated, "175 practice questions?!?" She confidently replied, "Yes, 175 questions." I then inquired, "How many questions do you think you should practice before a specialty board exam?" Her answer…"I don't know; 200 questions?" That was the problem! She did not know the appropriate preparation requirements.

I clearly stated the typical preparation requirements, "If you are going to read and complete questions, you need to go through one review book series, completely from start to finish *at least* once and answer and review the explanations to 1500 questions. If you choose to only practice questions and thoroughly review the explanations for each answer, you must answer and review the explanations to 2500 questions." The shocked look that had been on my face earlier apparently transferred to hers. I also recommended that when she read through the study material and/or questions that she write down everything she didn't know in a notebook that would become her study guide. This would help her be more active during her studying and when she went back to study the material again, she wouldn't waste time rereading the information she already knew. That study guide could then be pared down again with each review rewriting what she still didn't know into a smaller notebook.

We looked at when the next exam was scheduled (5 months away) and set up a study schedule that gave more time to areas that were more frequently tested and less time to areas on which she had performed well. At the end of each section, she was held accountable by having to bring her study notebook to me. We would then spend time discussing real patient cases that she had seen that reinforced the material she had just read and making sure she understood why and when and not just what or how. I was able to ask Dr. Kiersten to self-reflect on her progress and provide learner feedback on her work and effort. Sometimes, I will send the learner exam style questions that s/he must complete and return to me at the end of each section.

In this case the reassessment was clear and she was ready to retake the board exam. Several months ago, I received a thankful email from a proud Dr. Kiersten announcing that she had successfully passed the board examination.

2. Step-by-Step Approach to the Remediation of Clinical Skills

As with medical knowledge, the remediation of clinical skills tends to be one of the quickest processes. There are also many self-study resources available, either in textbooks, online modules or videos to aid with the remediation of clinical skills; however, it does require more resources and hands-on faculty teaching. It requires one-on-one mentoring in which the learner can practice performing the skills on real patients, standardized patients or through the use of simulators, and then receive constructive and corrective feedback. It may also require that you discuss some of the learner's prior barriers to learning these skills.

1. Meet with the Success Team to review the remediation plan, methods for learner reassessment and goals for successful remediation
   a. Program, course or clerkship director
   b. Faculty interested in leading the remediation
   c. The learner

2. Identify clinical skills gaps
    a. Review learner performance on prior clinical exams, standardized tests (OSCEs), observed mini or full clinical encounters (mini-CEX or CEX), simulations and written exams related to clinical skills
    b. Review her/his patient or procedure log to see what opportunities s/he has had in the clinical setting
    c. Is this problem new, global or specific to an isolated area of clinical skills?
    d. You may need to further observe the learner through clinical skills exams or direct observation to determine ongoing deficits or identify specific needs
3. Compare the learner's clinical skills gaps with the course requirements and identify where they overlap
4. Identify and document clinical skills goals for a given timeframe and review the expectations
5. Establish and communicate to the learner how s/he will be reassessed and what is required to pass the course
6. Assign reading, online modules or videos on physical exam skills or procedures, then consider assigning opportunities for the learner to observe others performing the procedure in real time
7. If possible, video record the learner practicing the deficient clinical skill
    a. Review the performance with the learner
    b. Ask the learner to self-assess her/his performance. Does s/he have insight?
    c. Point out any additional unidentified deficits to her/him (as well as strengths)
        i. Consider showing the learner a video of an outstanding or ideal example for comparison
    d. Give feedback and demonstrate missed elements with explanation of technique and reasoning behind each step of the technique
    e. Consider using standardized patients and simulators. Although somewhat contrived, they will allow the learner to practice her/his skills with an experienced 'patient' or practice model. Using these methods to encourage self-awareness and does not place a patient at risk of harm. These exercises can easily be video recorded and the learner can repeat the same exercise over and over as needed
8. Emphasize the need for repetition and practice
    a. Identify opportunities for practice outside of the clinical arena, such as practicing knot-tying at home or through video simulations

9. Look for evidence of improvement and provide feedback
   a. Continue to test learner on demonstration of missed skills
   b. Help the learner by confirming or refuting her/his exam findings or other clinical skills
   c. Emphasize the use of clinical reasoning as it relates to one's clinical skills
10. Learners can have their skills tested on a regular basis to determine the degree of improvement. An unbiased blinded third party can also compare the clinical skills exam performance (CEX) of the learner to her/his expected developmental level
11. Timely evaluations and feedback from clinical supervising physicians will also help measure the progress, as well as its sustainability

---

Example:

Upon notification by the director of the Foundations of Doctoring Course that a student, Rebecca, had failed her clinical assessment, she and I met with the director of the education assessment center. We reviewed her clinical exam scores and the video recorded portions of her exam to further identify her areas of weakness. She had a specific deficit in knowing when and how to perform the neurology exam. Other components of the exam and prior exams documented competence with other physical exam skills. Successful performance of each organ system exam was required to pass the course and the scheduled make-up exam was 3 weeks away.

Rebecca acknowledged that she ran out of time to study, having placed more priority on another exam and, in fact, was betting that she would be tested on the physical exam elements that she did have time to study.

Rebecca was assigned reading in a specific physical examination textbook and watching videos of the exam available through the library and her online curriculum. I re-reviewed her prior exam videos with her, so that she could self-assess her prior performance and talk about what she could do differently in the future. We then used a standardized patient on whom she practiced the exam. I observed and gave her feedback on her performance. We were also able to review the relevance of each exam element—when a clinician would use it and how to apply the information extracted. Rebecca demonstrated increasing confidence as she was given opportunities to practice clinical skills scenarios in the same format as the upcoming make-up exam. The student was also encouraged to practice the neurology exam as much as possible on friends and family and patients in her precepted continuity clinic.

With just a few interactions, Rebecca went from a failing student to one who received a perfect score on the make-up exam.

3. Step-by-Step Approach to the Remediation of Clinical Reasoning and Judgment

Compared to the prior 2 competencies, the remediation of clinical reasoning and judgment is by far the most labor intensive and time consuming. It requires that the student commit to daily reading and the independent completion of work on patient cases. It also takes ongoing faculty guidance and feedback at a high frequency of at least 3 times per week. These learners often have a lot of ground to make up, relative to their peers. Progress is slow and this can be frustrating because there is also a sense of urgency. This urgency comes from the learner's education timeline and, more importantly, patient safety concerns. With patience and concerted effort on both sides, success is achievable.

There are several great texts that examine how to teach and learn clinical reasoning; however, I have found that they are often too sophisticated and complex for the struggling learner who requires remediation. While this algorithm may seem overly simplistic, it has been very successful in the remediation of learners from student level to fellows. High level understanding and processing of clinical reasoning can follow, once these skills are mastered.

1. Meet with the Success Team to review the remediation plan, methods for learner reassessment and goals for successful remediation
   a. Program, course or clerkship director
   b. Faculty interested in leading the remediation
   c. The learner
2. To obtain a better understanding of the learner's strengths and weaknesses
   a. Ask the student to bring old history and physical exam write-ups and daily progress notes
   b. The faculty member should review the clinical reasoning involved in these old cases with the learner
   c. The faculty member should present unfamiliar cases on paper either with standardized patients or real patients, and assess the learner's ability to reason through a new case
   d. It may be helpful to identify the learner's heuristic errors to prevent premature closure. Ask yourself if they are making the same type of error over and over
      i. Anchoring bias—the initial impression was that it was one diagnosis and that is not changed despite new conflicting information

   ii. Availability bias—diagnosis chosen because it was recently seen and comes to mind easily
   iii. Gambling bias—if you flip a coin and get 10 heads in a row, the odds of getting heads again is still 50:50, so even if the learner has admitted 5 cases of congestive heart failure, the 6th case may also be congestive heart failure
   iv. Confirmation bias—Only places weight on information that confirms your diagnosis
3. Teach the learner a framework for creating a differential diagnosis. Here are 3 common frameworks
   a. Anatomical framework
      i. For example, what anatomical structures are in or refer to the right upper quadrant that could cause pain?
      ii. What are the structures of the eye and visual pathways that might result in blurry vision?
   b. Systems Approach
      i. Acronym RICHMOND

         R—Respiratory/Rheumatology
         I—Infectious Disease
         C—Cardiology
         H—Hematology
         M—Metabolic/Mental Health
         O—Oncology
         N—Neurology/Nephrology
         D—Digestive

      ii. Acronym VINDICATE AIDS

         V—Vascular
         I—Infectious
         N—Neoplastic
         D—Degenerative
         I—Inflammatory
         C—Congenital
         A—Autoimmune
         T—Traumatic
         E—Endocrinal and Metabolic
         A—Allergic
         I—Iatrogenic
         D—Drugs
         S—Social

   c. Pathophysiologic framework
      i. For example, in the work-up of anemia, it can be subdivided into macrocytic, normocytic or microcytic
4. Ask the learner to create differential diagnosis (DDx) based on a given age, gender, race/ethnicity and chief complaint
   a. Include most likely diagnoses AND the diagnoses that you don't want to miss
   b. List these 3–6 diagnoses
   c. Have the learner repeat this step, practicing with different presentations
      i. 50-year-old African American male with chest pain
      ii. 90-year-old Caucasian male with new onset seizures
      iii. 2-yearold Hispanic female with a rash and fever
   d. Resources such as First Consult can help the learner initiate a differential based on chief complaint and age that the learner can then customize to the given patient presentation
5. Ask the learner to identify relevant HPI questions and ROS questions by
   a. Collecting initial chronological information detailing the chief complaint
   b. Asking rule in or rule out questions for the 3–6 diagnoses on her/his differential diagnosis
   c. Repeating this step with the learner practicing with different presentations so that s/he can learn how to ask the most high yield questions
6. At first, provide the learner with feedback on Steps 4 and 5 and then direct your learner towards published references to self-correct for future cases
   a. Is her/his differential diagnosis appropriate?
   b. What questions did s/he remember to ask?
   c. What questions did s/he forget to ask?
   d. Is s/he asking too many extraneous questions?
   e. What additional information does s/he want to know from the patient?
   f. Ask the learner to reorder her/his differential or perhaps even add a diagnosis
7. Ask the learner to list physical exam elements that are both crucial (i.e. vital signs) in assessing the patient and that will help rule in or rule out the 3–6 diagnoses on her/his differential diagnosis
   a. Remind the learner that every element of the physical exam should be intentional so that he is alert and looking for specific information

   b. Require the learner to repeat this step of creating lists of physical exam elements with different case presentations
8. At first, provide feedback, and then for future cases direct your learner towards published references to check reasoning and judgment
   a. What PE elements did s/he remember to perform?
   b. What PE elements did s/he forget to perform?
   c. Is s/he performing too many extraneous exam elements?
   d. Ask the learner to reorder her/his differential or perhaps even add a diagnosis
9. Create a problem list
   a. The problem list should include every abnormal piece of information collected, including findings that are identified by standards as "normal" when they shouldn't be
      i. For example, a creatinine of 1.0mg/dL in a 90-year-old woman who weighs 55kg or a "normal" hematocrit in a chronically hypoxic patient
10. Encourage the learner to ask herself/himself these questions
   a. Have you seen a similar case before?
   b. Have you read about a similar case before?
   c. How is this case the same and how is it different? Compare and contrast!
   d. Analyze each diagnosis on the differential. What information (positive and negative) helps to rule in or rule out each of the diagnoses? Compare and contrast!
11. Give the learner a framework for choosing the diagnostic plan and review the case appropriate options
   a. Diagnostic framework
      i. Monitor the patient?
      ii. Order a lab?
      iii. Order a test?
      iv. Prescribe a medication?
   b. Have the student predict diagnostic outcomes, a simplistic way of getting at pre/post-test probabilities
      i. "I predict that the test will be normal; however, I think it is necessary to rule out a bacterial meningitis"
   c. Have the student reflect on consequences of her/his choices
      i. Patient risks, efficiency, too much data or not enough, etc
12. At first, provide feedback and then direct your learner towards published references with practice algorithms to confirm the appropriate work-up for future cases

   a. Which diagnostic elements did you correctly choose?
   b. Which diagnostic elements did you incorrectly choose and why?
   c. What are you missing and why?
13. Review treatment options including follow-up plans
   a. Have the learner predict the disease course without treatment
   b. Have the learner review treatment options
   c. Have learner anticipate the consequences of her/his treatment choices, including benefits and potential complications
   d. Have the learner state her/his final treatment recommendation as learning how to commit to one's beliefs is a crucial learning curve in medicine
14. Have the learner create an ongoing list of clinical questions to look up and apply to the care of her/his patients
15. Reinforce the use of additional resources, such as senior clinicians or consultants for feedback
   a. Use chart stimulated recall when providing feedback to your learner
16. On rounds and in clinic, the learner should be encouraged to explain her/his reasoning on major clinical decisions for additional feedback
   a. Errors in reasoning must be corrected immediately
   b. This will likely require some role modeling on the part of the mentor in the form of "thinking out loud." The learner should be encouraged to pay attention to how her/his colleagues present and formulate plans
   c. Especially for residents and more senior learners do not give the learner the plan if s/he is unable to develop one; rather teach her/him where to find the answer.
17. After establishing expectations, the learner's performance is best assessed by conversations with the supervising attendings/clinicians and having an unbiased faculty member conduct chart reviews with the learner
18. Residents with this difficulty may require a lighter patient load to have time to construct their reasoning

---

Example:

A resident, Jeannie, was sent to me by her residency director from another department for both diagnosis of the learner's deficit(s) and remediation. After my assessment, her greatest deficit was determined to be clinical reasoning. The residency program director, Jeannie and I sat down to discuss the outline for the remediation plan which included completing daily questions related to cases and meeting with me 3 times a week for one hour sessions to review the process of clinical reasoning. The goal was to transform Jeannie into an early manager within 8 weeks. Jeannie would be reassessed by completing a 2 week clinical block in which the faculty member and resident evaluators would be blinded to the resident's prior struggles.

While reviewing Jeannie's previously completed chart documentation, it was difficult for me to follow her thought process or to determine what strategies she used to approach clinical reasoning. Upon further questioning, Jeannie did not have a strategy. I started by teaching her the 3 possible frameworks for creating a differential and made recommendations as to when to use each of the 3 frameworks.

I then provided Jeannie with the age, gender, ethnicity and chief complaint of 6 cases. Jeannie was asked to go home and create 2 lists—a list of 3 to 5 of the most common diagnoses based on the information provided and a list of the top 3 diagnoses that you wouldn't want to miss. Jeannie was also asked to list the relevant history questions associated with each of the diagnoses listed. At the following meeting, we discussed the most prevalent diseases for each case and reviewed the questions. I then referred her to resources to look up such information, so that she could confirm her own clinical reasoning when I was not available to help.

Jeannie was sent home with the same cases and asked to create a list of the most clinically relevant physical exam elements to perform and why. She was asked to use resources to check her own clinical reasoning. At the next meeting, Jeannie was provided with additional information for each case, answering her history questions and providing the results of her requested physical exam elements. Together, we re-ordered the differential and I provided feedback on her progress and effort. A discussion ensued comparing and contrasting the diagnoses on the differential.

At the next meeting, she brought a list of her proposed diagnostic work-up and treatments for each of the cases, cross-referenced and checked through a review of the literature. We discussed the diagnostic work-up choices and treatment options, along with the anticipated outcomes. The process was repeated with a different set of cases, this time all with the same chief complaint to emphasize the importance of subtlety and comparing and contrasting.

While on rounds, Jeannie has been instructed to spend more time explaining her reasoning and she has asked her attending to encourage this verbalization. Specifically, she decided to use the SNAPPS method of presentation (see **Table 8.3**), which stands for:

S—Summarize history and findings
N—Narrow the differential to 2–3 most likely
A—Analyze the differential by comparing and contrasting
P—Plan treatment and further work-up
P—Probe the preceptor about uncertainties and alternatives
S—Select an issue related to the care for self-directed learning

TABLE 8.3 Written H&P, Written SOAP Note, and Presentation Templates for Emphasizing and Practicing Clinical Reasoning and Judgment. These templates can also be used for those who struggle with time management and organization.

Written History and Physical Template

Date: **Time:**

Chief Complaint:

History of Present Illness:

- Paragraph 1
  1. Starts: "Mr/s. (name) is a (age) year old (race/ethnicity) (gender) with a past medical history of (up to 4 elements from PmHx, SocHx, FmHx, that are relevant to the current chief complaint) presents with…(chief complaint)
  2. Describe patient's symptoms chronologically
  3. Consider top 4 possible diagnoses
- Paragraph 2
  1. State the symptoms and review of systems findings that support or refute your top 4 hypotheses
  2. State the presence or absence of risk factors that support or refute your top 4 hypotheses

Past Medical History:

- List all diseases, surgeries, immunizations, pregnancies/deliveries, developmental history, hospitalizations
- Include dates and indicators of disease severity when possible
- Cross-check list with medication list to make sure the list includes all diagnoses for which the patient is taking medicine

Medications:

- List all prescription medications using the generic name, with doses and route
- List all over the counter medications, vitamins and herbal supplements

Allergies:

- List cause and reaction

Family History:

- List all illnesses, deaths, surgeries of at least the first degree relatives
- May acknowledge healthy relatives

(continued)

Written History and Physical Template (continued)

Social History:

- Occupation/schooling
- Exposures (tobacco, alcohol, illicit drugs, work, travel exposures, animal exposures, as appropriate)
- With whom do they live
- Who assists them and in what capacity
- State the Primary Care Provider

Review of Systems:

- Ask questions about each of the following systems as it relates to the clerkship/rotation
    1. General/Constitutional
    2. Skin/Breast
    3. Eyes/Ears/Nose/Mouth/Throat
    4. Cardiovascular
    5. Respiratory
    6. Gastrointestinal
    7. Genitourinary
    8. Musculoskeletal
    9. Neurologic/Psychiatric
    10. Allergic/Immunologic/Lymphatic/Endocrine

Physical Exam:

- Do a complete physical exam
- Start with general appearance and vitals, then proceed thorough all systems
- Included pertinent positive and negative findings

Data:

- List most recent laboratory data with accompanying baseline data if different from current
- List most recent radiological data with comparison to prior imaging when available
- List recent microbiology data, if available
- List other data, i.e. EKGs, ECHOs, PFTs, Stress Tests

Problem List:

- Not for presentation, just to organize thoughts
- List all established diagnoses, symptoms, abnormal vitals, abnormal physical exam signs, collected data

(continued)

Written History and Physical Template (continued)

Assessment:

- This is a summary statement of key H&P elements
- Start with the following: Mr/s (name) is a (age) year old (race/ethnicity) (gender) with a past medical history of (up to 4 diseases, developmental history elements, social history, family history that relate directly to the chief complaint) presents with (chief complaint) and was found to have (positive and pertinent negative findings from history, physical, and data)

Plan:

- Order your problems from most active to least active
- For each element on the problem list
  1. Symptom or Diagnosis from problem list
     A. Differential diagnosis (top 3 or 4). If the diagnosis is well established, such as Type 2 DM, then your differential can be controlled vs. uncontrolled
     B. State evidence leaning toward each diagnosis, evidence against diagnosis
     C. Diagnostic plan—monitor, order a lab, order a test, order a medication
     D. Treatment plan and follow-up
  2. Symptom or Diagnosis from problem list: etc…

Signature with name written in print or stamped, followed by title or as per the electronic medical record

Written SOAP Note Template

Date: **Time:**

History of Present Illness:

- Paragraph 1
  1. Starts: "Mr/s. (name) is a (age) year old (race/ethnicity) (gender) with a past medical history of (up to 4 elements from PmHx, SocHx, FmHx that are relevant to the current chief complaint) presents with…(chief complaint).
  2. Describe patient's symptoms chronologically
  3. Consider top 3–5 possible diagnoses
- Paragraph 2
  1. State the symptoms and review of systems findings that support or refute your top 3–5 hypotheses

(continued)

Written SOAP Note Template (continued)

2. State the presence or absence of risk factors that support or refute your top 3–5 hypotheses. Risk factors can be from PmHx, Meds, Allergies, FmHx, SocHx

Physical Exam:

- Start with general appearance and vitals, then proceed thorough pertinent systems
- Included pertinent positive and negative findings

Data (if available and pertinent):

- List recent laboratory data with accompanying baseline data
- List recent radiological data with comparison to prior imaging when available
- List recent microbiology data
- List other data, i.e. EKGs, ECHOs, PFTs, Stress Tests

Problem List (optional):

- Not for presentation, just to organize thoughts
- List all established diagnosis, symptoms, abnormal vitals, abnormal physical exam signs, collected data

Assessment:

- This is a summary statement of key H&P elements
- Start with the following: Mr/s (name) is a (age) year old (race/ethnicity) (gender) with a past medical history of (up to 4 diseases, developmental history elements, social history, family history that relate directly to the chief complaint) presents with (chief complaint) and was found to have (positive and negative findings from history, physical, and data)

Plan:

- Order your problems from most active to least active
- For each element on the problem list
    1. Symptom or Diagnosis from problem list
        A. Differential diagnosis (top 3 or 4). If the diagnosis is well established, such as Type 2 DM, then your differential can be controlled vs. uncontrolled
        B. State evidence leaning toward each diagnosis, evidence against diagnosis, or how the patient meets criteria for controlled vs. not controlled
        C. Diagnostic plan—monitor, order a lab, order a test, order a medication
        D. Treatment plan and follow-up
    2. Symptom or Diagnosis from problem list: etc…

Signature with name written in print or stamped, followed by title or as per the electronic medical record

Presentation Template

The presentation is not a regurgitation of the H&P. It is a more focused and concise format. The SNAPPS model is recommended.

S—Summarize the history and findings

- HPI: "Mr/s. (name) is a (age) year old (race/ethnicity) (gender) with a past medical history of (up to 4 elements from PmHx, SocHx, FmHx that are relevant to the current chief complaint) presents with…(chief complaint)
- Describe patient's symptoms chronologically
- State the review of systems findings that support or refute your top 4 hypotheses. (Do not explicitly state hypotheses)
- PMHx, Meds/All, FmHx, SocHx: Include everything from the H&P that you need to think about/worry about during the hospitalization, group them by category
- Physical Exam: Organize your findings by system. Include the positive and negative findings that are related to your most likely diagnosis. Include any other significant or abnormal exam findings.
- Diagnostic tests: Report labs and studies that argue for or against the most likely diagnoses (save your hypotheses and reasoning for later). State any other abnormal labs or studies which you need to think about

N—Narrow the differential

- Verbalize the top 2–3 most likely diagnoses for each problem or group of problems
- Order the list from most to least likely

A—Analyze the differential

- Compare and contrast the possible diagnoses by stating the evidence for and against each diagnostic possibly on your list as it relates to the case
- Discuss discriminating findings
- Verbalize your thinking process

P—Probe the preceptor

- Ask your preceptor questions about any uncertainties, difficulties, or alternative approaches
- Reveal areas of confusion
- The preceptor has a knowledge base and clinical reasoning skills that can be readily accessed

P—Plan management:

- Initiate a discussion of the patient management plan per problem, this may be diagnostic, therapeutic, or both
- Be as brief and specific as possible
- Repeat the N, A, P, P for each problem or group of problems

S—Select case-related issue for self-study

- Commit to learning about focused, patient-based questions

(continued)

Presentation Template (continued)

Additional Recommendations:

1. Approximate timing for oral presentations:

History of present illness	1 min
PMHx, Meds/All, SocHx, FmHx	45–60 sec
Physical Exam	60–75 sec
Data	30–45 sec
Assessment, Plan	4–5 min

2. When you start working with a new attending, you may show them these templates and ask if you can use this format. It will give the attending a chance to communicate expectations and identify any differences unique to the rotation or to their preferences.

She also requested feedback from her attending physicians. At the end of the remediation, she was reassessed on a subsequent rotation where the evaluator was unaware of her prior need for remediation.

Jeannie mailed me a copy of her passing evaluation, including average scores in clinical reasoning! She has since completed residency with no further concerns regarding her clinical reasoning and no reported patient safety concerns.

Table 8.3 provides 3 templates that can be used for teaching the clinical reasoning process around documenting and for presenting the H&P and SOAP notes.

Learners who have difficulty understanding how to ask patients effective questions can practice playing the 1940s parlor game of twenty questions on non-medical topics. This idea comes from Debra Klamen, MD and Reed G. Williams, PhD's book on standardized patient exam failures. Twenty questions encourages deductive clinical reasoning and creativity. Choose a subject but do not reveal it to the learner. The learner then asks up to twenty yes or no questions until they identify the subject or run out of questions. Discuss her/his approach with her/him. Is it organized? Is it efficient? Were all of her/his questions high yield? Discuss the game's correlation to the process of medical history taking.

Blankenburg R. et al. wrote a resource that I find particularly helpful entitled, "Revisiting How We Think: Innovative Ideas for Promoting and Assessing Clinical Reasoning." While they give many techniques for improving clinical reasoning, some of my favorites include asking the learner to highlight the pertinent positive and negative elements within the history, physical, and data sections, based on her/his leading diagnoses. This requires learners to highlight their reasoning as they flow through a patient encounter.

Blankenburg R. et al. also ask the learner to create charts to assist with clinical reasoning. I will often ask the learner to choose one presentation and then create a generic (not patient-specific) chart that lists symptoms and history, signs and data unique to each diagnosis on the differential to allow for comparing and contrasting. The charts recommended by Blankenburg et al. are even more inclusive, with rows for epidemiology, pathophysiology, treatment, etc. The last technique I use, which is also similar to Blankenburg's, is to have the learner weigh the significance of the pertinent positives and negatives in relation to a patient specific differential through a concrete chart (see **Table. 8.4**).

Sometimes, when initiating a remediation plan, you may choose the "wrong" deficit to remediate. However, further work with the learner will quickly illuminate the problem. Take the example of a surgical resident who kept getting into trouble for making poor clinical decisions. On the first day of remediation, I realized that the problem wasn't his clinical decision making, but rather an undiagnosed

TABLE 8.4 Sample Charts to Aid with the Remediation of Clinical Reasoning and Judgment

Presenting Symptom: Chest Pain	Symptoms and historical info.	Signs	Data
GERD	Subacute, epigastric, burning, supine, relief with antacids	Tenderness to palpation of the epigastrium	Abnormal EGD
Stable Angina	Male, pressure with radiation to arm or jaw, exertional, +/-SOB, nausea, DM, HTN, HLD, tobacco, FmHx	May have murmur, lateral PMI, gallop, paradox split S2, or normal	Abnormal EKG, Dynamic EKG
Etc.			

	Epigastric	Not exertional	Burning	S4
GERD	↑↑	↑↑	↑↑	↓
Stable Angina	↓	↓↓	↓	↑
Etc.				

impairment of his vision. The key was that all of his "clinical reasoning" errors occurred while making patient assessments with a binocular microscope.

4. Step-by-Step Approach to the Remediation of Time Management and Organization

Most learners respond readily to direction and suggestions regarding time management and organization. This skill is very teachable. Most of our learners just need structure and practical tools as they have never been asked to manage so much information and to multitask at this high level before.

1. Meet with the Success Team to review the remediation plan, methods for learner reassessment and goals for successful remediation
   a. Program, course or clerkship director
   b. Faculty interested in leading the remediation
   c. The learner
2. Have the learner think about how the lack of organization is preventing competent performance and link the two together for the learner if necessary
3. Review the overall expectations with your learner
   a. Identify how much you expect the learner to accomplish in a given time frame
      i. "You should be able to write a follow-up note in 15 minutes or less."
      ii. "You have 15 minutes to review the old records. Think about where you should look first to find the most important information or a summary of information"
      iii. "You should be able to see 8 patients this afternoon and have the notes completed by 6PM at the latest"
4. Obtain the learner's perspective and concerns
   a. Is this a new problem? Does this struggle also exist in her/his personal life? What strategies does s/he use in her/his personal life, and do they work?
   b. Are there specific things preventing organization or efficiency?
   c. What methods is s/he using or has s/he tried to improve this deficit?
   d. What methods has s/he observed in her/his peers or seniors that help with time management and organization?
5. Teach one data organization system
   a. A check-box to-do list (This is the most common system)
   b. A to-do list at the bottom of each progress note

   c. A to-do list on the prior shift's sign-out sheet
   d. An H&P or note template
   e. A list of the day's patients to be seen or a daily outline
6. After the learner has created her/his data organization system for the morning, day, week, etc. review the tasks to be completed with the learner
   a. Did s/he record all of them? Add missing tasks. Eliminate unnecessary tasks
   b. Were any tasks misunderstood or misinterpreted?
7. Help the learner prioritize the list of tasks
   a. Highlight what needs to be done first
   b. Star the items of highest priority
   c. Reorder the list as needed
   d. Include time periods
      i. "This must be done in the next 2 hours"
      ii. "Be sure to call all consults before lunch"
8. Model the behavior you wish to see
   a. For example, observe the learner and then model pre-rounding in the hospital setting, or chart reviewing in the clinic
      i. Demonstrate how to collect information in a quick systematic way
      ii. Have your learner use the same method for pre-rounding or chart review with every patient to save time through repetition and to ensure thoroughness
      iii. Plan the patient encounter before walking in the room. After asking the patient how they are doing, what are the key questions that you need answered based on the history and presentation? Know that the learner can go back, call or see the patient again at a later time or date for more information. Flexibility with patient encounters will come after one has mastered efficiency
9. Consider having the learner keep a minute-to-minute log of daily activities or 30 minute log for the week
   a. Identify where time is being lost
   b. Identify ways of increasing efficiency with different tasks
10. Have the learner observe and discuss time management and organization strategies with her/his peers and seniors
11. Provide the learner with both reinforcing and corrective feedback
12. The learner may need a lighter patient load at first to complete a day's work or graduated decreasing time constraints
    a. For example, you have 90 minutes to collect the H&P this week and 60 minutes next week, or you have 10 minutes to present your patient

this week and 8 minutes the following week with a goal of getting your presentations down to 5 minutes

13. The learner's performance is best assessed by Mini-CEXs, conversations with the supervising faculty and residents and sign-in and sign-out times
14. Limit unnecessary disruptions
    a. If you work in a multi-site system, try to keep the learner at the same site for multiple consecutive rotations so they can work on efficiency without having to learn new systems in the process
15. Time management can become very stressful as the learner struggles to complete tasks within a reasonable amount of time and is often unprepared for rounds, despite working longer days
    a. Stress management should be emphasized
    b. Suggestions should be made for managing stress
    c. An evaluation from an outside professional is recommended. If the learner is requiring remediation, this is a large enough stressor to warrant an evaluation

---

Example:

A medical student, Greg, was struggling to organize his day while working on an inpatient rotation. The clerkship block director and I met with Greg to discuss our concerns. He admitted feeling overwhelmed and was quite relieved that we were offering to help. The daily expectations were reviewed with him so that he knew what had to be organized and completed each day. For example, Greg was to spend 30 minutes pre-rounding on each patient and "skeletonize" his notes, 5 minutes to present each patient, 15 minutes to write orders and call consults on each patient, an additional 15–20 minutes to complete each note and then spend the rest of the day following up on tasks and revisiting patients.

I modeled how to pre-round in under 30 minutes per patient and then Greg was encouraged to use the same system every day to help increase his pace, while not missing anything. He was taught to create a check-box list of things to do while on rounds and to cross-check the list with his resident who used the same system. This cross-checking was essential to make sure that he had not missed any tasks. The resident was then able to tell Greg which patient orders had to be entered first.

Greg caught on quickly. Had he not, I would have spent the morning with him, watching and modeling ways to be more efficient, as I have for other students. Greg also sought feedback from his resident and attending physicians, who both noticed a dramatic improvement in his ability to accomplish tasks in a timely manner. He reported being less stressed and no longer needing to stay in the hospital into the evenings to finish his work.

On subsequent rotation evaluations, he scored highly in time management, efficiency and organization.

Example:

CJ, a physician assistant student, was having difficulty organizing his daily notes. Specifically, the information in the history of present illness and assessment and plan sections seemed sporadic and were hard to follow.

He was specifically told to use the following method as described in Table 8.3 and place in a template in **Table 8.5** to structure the history of present illness information:

- Paragraph 1
  1. Starts: "Mr/s. (name) is a (age) year old (race/ethnicity) (gender) with a past medical history of (up to 4 elements from PmHx, SocHx, FmHx that are relevant to the current chief complaint) presents with …(chief complaint)
  2. Describe patient's symptoms chronologically
  3. Consider top 4 possible diagnoses, but do not include them in the written documentation
- Paragraph 2
  1. State the symptoms and review of systems findings that support or refute your top 4 hypotheses
  2. State the presence or absence of risk factors that support or refute your top 4 hypotheses

Once he mastered this, which took about 1 week, he was told to use the following method to structure the assessment and plan section:

Assessment:

- This is a summary statement of key H&P elements
- Start with the following: Mr/s (name) is a (age) year old (race/ethnicity) (gender) with a past medical history of (up to 4 diseases, developmental history elements, social history, family history that relate directly to the chief complaint) presents with (chief complaint) and was found to have (positive and negative findings from history, physical and data)

Plan:

- Order your problems from most active to least active

- For each element on the problem list
  1. First symptom or diagnosis from problem list
     a. Differential diagnosis (top 3 or 4)
     b. State evidence leaning toward each diagnosis and evidence against diagnosis
     c. Diagnostic plan—which may include monitoring, a lab, a test, or a diagnostic treatment
     d. Treatment plan—which may include medication, monitoring, follow-up, patient education, etc.
  2. Second symptom or diagnosis from problem list: as above
  3. Etc.

Within 3 weeks, CJ's performance had dramatically improved. Working with his notes was less of a challenge and he passed the rotation.

TABLE 8.5 Template to Fill in While Collecting Information About a Patient Encounter. Some of the details may vary based on specialty to include information such as birth history, immunization or pregnancy history.

History and Physical Template To Fill In

Date: **Time:**

CC:

HPI:

______________________ is a ___ year old ________ ________

with a PMHX of ___________ who presents with:

Chronology

____

____

____

Pertinent + and –

____

____

____

(continued)

TABLE 8.5 Template to Fill in While Collecting Information About a Patient Encounter (continued)

History and Physical Template To Fill In

Past Medical History:

Diseases

____

____

Surgeries

____

____

Medications:

____

____

____

Allergies:

____

____

Family History:

Illnesses

____

Premature Deaths

____

Social History:

Occupation/schooling

____

Exposures

____

Living situation

____

PCP

____

(continued)

TABLE 8.5 Template to Fill in While Collecting Information About a Patient Encounter (continued)

History and Physical Template To Fill In

Review of Systems:

____

____

____

____

Physical Exam:

Vitals

____

____

Pertinent Findings

____

____

Data:

Labs

____

Micro

____

Radiology

____

Other

____

Assessment:

Summary statement

____

____

____

____

____

(continued)

TABLE 8.5 Template to Fill in While Collecting Information About a Patient Encounter (continued)

History and Physical Template To Fill In
Plan:
Active Problem
A. DDx
B. Evidence for DDx
C. Diagnostic plan
D. Treatment plan and Follow-up
Active Problem
A. DDx
B. Evidence for DDx
C. Diagnostic plan
D. Treatment plan and Follow-up
Active Problem
A. DDx
B. Evidence for DDx
C. Diagnostic plan
D. Treatment plan and Follow-up
Non-Active Problem
A. Treatment plan and Follow-up
Non-Active Problem
A. Treatment plan and Follow-up

Example:

Gretchen was a brilliant MD, PhD resident who had a love for detail. While at times this was a great asset, she kept falling behind in clinic. She would spend much more time than was allotted for each patient. She would walk in and begin collecting all information—pertinent and unrelated—and then try to organize all of the information after she left the patient's room. I instructed her to take a look at the reason for the patient's visit and try to come up with key questions prior to entering the room. After asking the patient how they are feeling, double check that your questions are appropriate and then limit yourself to just a few key questions. Here was her response…

> *"I wanted to send you an update on my progress in clinic. Like we talked about, I've been preparing approximately 5 questions ahead of time for patients whose complaint I know ahead of time. I think that's gone really well and it's given me a different frame of mind about history-taking. Namely, I now*

feel like once I've asked the questions I feel are important, I'm done. This has really helped me get through things faster because before I just felt like I had to exhaust all the questions I could think of.

We also talked about patients who come up with a new complaint in the room. I was supposed to just ask questions that specifically ruled in/out possible diagnoses. I have to say I haven't been as systematic about that but I feel like it's still gotten a lot better. I ask just what I think are the most important things and then move on. I checked in again with my preceptor who feels like I'm doing much better. I really appreciate your help and, like I said, I really think that your suggestions have made a big difference. Thank you."

5. Step-by-Step Approach to the Remediation of Interpersonal Skills

All faculty are responsible for modeling this skill set for their learners.

Role modeling, increased supervision, addressing the underlying cause and an official warning letter/probation are the most effective ways of managing this subset of deficiencies. Further assistance with a mental health evaluation and treatment when indicated is strongly recommended. If you get frustrated with the learner, think deficit not defiance. Compassion works better than authoritarian confrontation.

1. Meet with the Success Team to review the remediation plan, methods for learner reassessment and goals for successful remediation
    a. Program, course or clerkship director
    b. Faculty interested in leading the remediation
    c. The learner
2. Ask the learner to identify *and* commit the following to writing: how interpersonal skills and collaboration throughout the workday can either facilitate or hinder patient care
    a. If s/he needs a framework for her/his response, you may give her/him one, i.e., with patients, with patient families, with colleagues, with supervising doctors, with nurses and other staff
3. Review the relevance of good interpersonal skills
    a. Expand upon what the learner brings to you
    b. Discuss with the learner how the lack of good interpersonal skills is preventing competent performance
4. Identify what you expect the learner to accomplish in a given time frame
5. Be prepared with examples of specific conflicts or interpersonal challenges that your learner has faced

   a. Give examples of reported interpersonal skills deficiencies or conflicts
   b. Address directly and privately
   c. Give the learner a chance to reply and discuss
   d. Talk about overall goals, perspectives, and perceptions related to the example
   e. Have the learner self-reflect
   f. Have the learner provide or model alternative examples of how they could have reacted in the same situation
   g. Have the learner consider the wishes and needs of others (patient, nurse, etc.) and her/his perspectives in the conflict and with the alternative examples
6. Videotape interactions as appropriate to facilitate self-awareness
7. Have the learner identify a role model with good interpersonal skills that s/he would want to emulate. Make sure that it is someone you feel would serve as a good role model
8. Consider a mental health evaluation/referral
   a. Most states have physician health programs (www.fsphp.org), or consider services through the learner's insurance
9. Discuss academic consequences of poor behaviors
   a. Letter of warning or focused review
   b. Probation, including future repercussions of needing to disclose probationary status throughout her/his career
   c. Difficulty obtaining letters of recommendation for next stage of career
10. Discuss the career consequences
   a. Monitoring by the licensing board
   b. If put on probation, s/he will need to explain it throughout her/his career
   c. Frequent job turnover
   d. Fewer patient referrals
   e. Lower income
   f. Less stability and job satisfaction
11. Increased supervision to monitor interactions and provide feedback
12. Supervising faculty evaluations can be used to measure progress. 360 degree evaluations, including patient evaluations, may be indicated.

Example:

A fellow, Darren, was referred to the remediation program because he was intermittently rude to the nursing staff when they paged him and abrupt with his colleagues if they came to him with work that would lengthen his workday. He was referred for remediation of poor interpersonal skills. Upon further discussion, Darren had tremendous insight into his behavior. He acknowledged that at times he was rude to others and that it happened when he was feeling most stressed. He also knew and admitted that he needed to improve to provide the best possible patient care.

Self-awareness in this case was not the issue. While most learners struggling with interpersonal skills are defensive and require a certain amount of external pressure to change their behavior, he acquiesced and therefore the step-by-step approach was tailored to his individual needs.

Example continued...

I inquired further into why he was most stressed at the end of the day and learned that he had a sick family member at home who depended on him for activities of daily living, including bathing, cooking and household chores. The fellow was offered a leave of absence which he didn't know was an option. After the family member passed away, the complaints of poor interpersonal skills disappeared.

Of note, as with professionalism deficits, the learner is much more likely to succeed with remediation if you are able to identify an underlying cause.

Example:

Just recently, a second year resident was having difficulty assuming his new role as a leader on the inpatient team. Having been a very good intern, Cole would revert to the role of an intern rather than work to master his new position. He had difficulty interacting with the team and knowing what he should be doing as a supervising resident. Many learners remember what their residents did for them, what they liked and what they would not want to emulate. Others need more explicit instruction. To that end, I created this checklist which he and others have been using successfully (see **Table 8.6**).

TABLE 8.6 A Sample Checklist of Resident Responsibilities

Resident Team Leader Role

Day 1

1. Verbally review your expectations with the team, addressing the role of each member
   - Can also provide written expectations
   - Include pre-rounding time, that all team members should see all of their patients and collect data prior to rounds, when and where to check in before rounds and at the end of the day
   - How much supervision to expect and when others should page you
   - Expectations regarding teaching frequency and timing
   - Bidirectional feedback weekly
   - Let each one know you will individualize her/his teaching based on how you think you can help her/him succeed
2. Ask the team members what their goals are
3. Review your expectations and personal goals with your attending

Daily

1. Pre-round on your patients, specifically be sure to visit or at least lay eyes on every patient as junior team members can have difficulty determining sick vs. not sick
   - Address any issues that cannot wait until rounds
2. Meet with the team approximately 10 minutes prior to rounds to discuss the plans that will be presented
3. During rounds, speak up after each patient to say you agree, disagree or elaborate on the presentation just given
4. Immediately after rounds, review your interns' and students' to-do lists
   - Ensure that they are complete
   - Help them prioritize the lists, i.e. what needs to happen before lunch
5. Complete your work, i.e. d/c summaries
6. Double check to make sure the interns are completing their tasks, usually by reviewing charts/medical records
7. View all patients to be admitted by the intern and medical students
   - Ensure they are stable prior to giving them to the juniors on the team
   - Place any necessary early orders to enhance timely patient care
8. Review each case with the resident or student after each has done a more thorough H&P and written orders
9. Afternoon rounds to review day's updates and teach 3–30 minutes depending on the day

Weekly

1. Get and give feedback to your team members

6. Step-by-Step Approach to the Remediation of Communication

On the University of Colorado campus, there is a Center for Advancing Professional Excellence that provides an environment for students to practice various clinical encounters with standardized patients as they would on clinical rotations. This resource comes with some cost and faculty time but it has been invaluable. It provides the learner an opportunity to practice the same encounter multiple times in an environment where he is free to learn from her/his mistakes and provide an opportunity for the learner to watch her/his communication skills via video recording of each patient encounter.

1. Meet with the Success Team to review the remediation plan, methods for learner reassessment and goals for successful remediation
   a. Program or clerkship director
   b. Faculty interested in leading the remediation
   c. The learner
2. Ask learner to identify *and* commit the following to writing
   a. How communication throughout the workday can either facilitate or hinder patient care
   b. If s/he needs a framework for her/his response, you may give her/him one i.e. with patients, with patient families, with colleagues, with supervising doctors, with nurses and other staff
3. Review the relevance of good communication skills and expectations with the learner
   a. Expand upon what the learner brings to you
   b. Discuss with the student how the lack of good communication is preventing competent performance
4. Identify what you expect the learner to accomplish in a given time frame
5. Assign reading from a communications textbook
6. Role model what you expect of your learner
   a. So that your learner knows what to focus on, consider having the learner use the Calgary-Cambridge Observation Guide or similar guide while watching you, her/his preceptor or other faculty
7. Consider having the learner take or repeat communications classes or social skills classes
   a. Usually given during the first 2 years of medical school or non-clinical training
   b. Provided at local universities or in community education classes or Toastmasters (www.toastmaster.org)

   c. Programs offered by outside organizations for health professionals such as the Bayer Workshops in New Haven, Connecticut
8. Have the learner practice
   a. Oral presentations emphasizing strong clinical reasoning and organization and provide feedback
   b. Summarizing complex cases and give her/him feedback
   c. Specific skills with standardized patients
      i. Giving bad news
      ii. Interview about sensitive topic
      iii. Ask questions
9. View video recorded performances with the learner
   a. To augment self-awareness
   b. If using standardized patients, give feedback and repeat the same case to see if the learner can incorporate the feedback given
10. Teach the learner to clarify communication throughout her/his day
    a. Have the learner repeat back what is said
    b. Give her/him permission to ask for clarification
    c. Have her/him request direct language by telling her/his team and colleagues if s/he struggles with colloquial speech or slang
11. Private feedback should be given promptly throughout the workday
    a. To provide the most useful constructive criticism
    b. To assure that there is clear communication between the struggling learner and her/his patients and colleagues
    c. To allow the learner to ask follow-up questions after verbal interactions to make sure that the appropriate message was conveyed
12. Supervising faculty evaluations can be used to measure progress
    360 degree evaluations, including patient evaluations, may be indicated

---

Example:

A medical student, Jeff, was struggling with communication skills. The clerkship block director, the communication specialist and I met with Jeff to discuss our concerns and he was relieved that we were offering help. He had struggled his entire life with communication and social interactions. His fear of stuttering had left him a quiet observer, with little practice speaking. The expectations were reviewed with her/him so that he knew the plan for remediation and how his success would be measured.

Jeff was assigned reading from a communication textbook and was asked to complete the Calgary-Cambridge Observation Guide while watching faculty interact with patients. The communication specialist and I observed his interactions with standardized patients. It quickly became clear that the student was highly intelligent and had great clinical reasoning skills. As for his communication, it was very clear that he lacked rapport with his patients. He was given reinforcing and corrective feedback and was instructed to respond to the patient's statements instead of moving on to his agenda. There was a remarkable improvement. He was also encouraged to make eye contact and use more facial expressions. We watched the video records of his performance and he was surprised to see that he barely stuttered and, when he did, it was not at all distracting from his communication.

He also practiced presenting patient cases, as well as summarizing cases. He was offered a temporary tutor who would be available in the mornings for her/him to practice his presentations prior to rounds.

Subsequent faculty evaluations noted good communication skills. He went on to present in front of a large audience at a regional academic conference, during which he interacted with the audience and spoke with smooth speech.

Teach reciprocity by asking the learner to respond to the comments and actions of others in a similar manner. Learners may also benefit from reading about emotional and social intelligence. Empathy can be learned even if not felt through empathic social protocols that are internalized and implemented.

Cultural sensitivity training may be needed if the learner is from a different country, state or different socioeconomic background. Learners from other cultures may need to be explicitly told how their new community expects them to act. This might include handshakes, eye contact, direct questioning, smiling and acknowledging others' comments and concerns. Speech and language pathologists can help with accent modification. Also remember that for many of our young learners, the medical culture is a foreign culture even if they grew up in the same geographic community.

7. Step-by-Step Approach to the Remediation of Professionalism

For the remediation of professionalism, there are skeptics and idealists. While I prefer to be eternally optimistic, this is a tough problem. We all go through periods of time in our lives when we could act more professionally and these are considered minor lapses. Say for example, you are a male and you overslept this morning, didn't have time to shave and arrive at work with more than a 5PM shadow. You do not appear as clean cut as you would like given your professional role; however, this minor lapse does not interfere significantly with learning, the clinician-patient relationship or functioning of the health care team.

There are a small subset of learners whose unprofessional behavior *does* interfere significantly with learning, the clinician-patient relationship or functioning of the health care team. These are the learners who need remediation. When a learner has a major lapse, first ask yourself why would a reasonable person do this?

The common belief is that unprofessional behavior to this extent never goes away but can be kept at bay for months, years or even decades. Papadakis et al. found that unprofessional behavior in medical school, particularly being irresponsible or demonstrating minimal improvement, is strongly associated with subsequent disciplinary action among physicians by the state medical boards. Often, though, poor professionalism and work avoidance is based on a lack of skills, including medical knowledge, confidence and/or clinical reasoning. These undesirable attitudes are easier to change, because they naturally improve with improved skills. If you are able to identify an underlying cause, the learner is much more likely to succeed with remediation.

As with interpersonal skills deficits, think deficit not defiance. Compassion works better than authoritarian confrontation.

1. Meet with the Success Team to review the remediation plan, methods for learner reassessment and goals for successful remediation
    a. Program, course or clerkship director
    b. Faculty interested in leading the remediation
    c. The learner
2. Insight is essential! Ask them to write about the following topics. It may take time, but eventually you will see your learner evolve and develop her/his professional identity
    a. Reflect on her/his own level of professionalism
        i. Writing gives her/him a chance to process the concerns and to commit
        ii. Provides documentation for her/his file
    b. Ask the learner to identify *and* commit the following to writing: how professionalism throughout the workday can either facilitate or hinder patient care
        i. If he needs a framework for her/his response, you may give her/him one, i.e., with patients, with patient families, with colleagues, with supervising doctors, with nurses and other staff
3. Review the relevance of professionalism
    a. Expand upon what the learner brings to you

   b. Discuss with the learner how the lack of professionalism is preventing competent performance
   c. Discuss whether "physicians/clinicians need to suspend self-interest"
4. Identify what you expect the learner to accomplish in a given time frame
   a. Verbally and in writing, set strict behavioral guidelines and appropriate interpersonal boundaries
   b. State verbally and in writing what is not acceptable behavior
   c. Emphasize high level of accountability
   d. Document for the learner the consequences of poor professional behavior
5. Be prepared with examples of poor professionalism as displayed by the learner
   a. Give examples of reported poor professionalism
   b. Address directly and privately
   c. Give the learner a chance to reply and discuss
   d. Talk about overall goals, perspectives and perceptions related to the example
   e. Have the learner provide alternatives to her/his behavior in that situation. If unable verbally, have her/him think about it and send it to you in writing
   f. Have the learner self-reflect
6. Have the learner identify a role model that s/he would like to emulate and who you agree would serve as a good role model of professionalism
7. Videotape interactions as appropriate to facilitate self-awareness
8. Consider mental health evaluation/referral
   a. Most states have physician health programs (www.fsphp.org) or consider services through the learner's insurance
9. Discuss academic consequences of poor behaviors
   a. Letter of warning or focused review
   b. Probation, including future repercussions of needing to disclose probationary status throughout her/his career
   c. Difficulty obtaining letters and recommendations for next stage of career
10. Discuss the career consequences
    a. Monitoring by the licensing board
    b. If put on probation, s/he will need to explain it throughout her/his career
    c. Frequent job turnover
    d. Fewer patient referrals

   e. Lower income
   f. Less stability and job satisfaction
11. Increased supervision to monitor professionalism, ensure strict enforcement of the guidelines and provide feedback. Be prepared to follow through on documented consequences of poor professional behavior
12. For assessment to measure progress consider
    a. Supervising faculty evaluations
    b. 360 degree evaluations, including patient evaluations
    c. Arrival and departure times
    d. Attendance
    e. Professionalism reports
    f. Attire and appearance
13. Role modeling and an official letter of warning/probation are most effective. Limit setting may also be required by placing stipulations on electives choices, moonlighting and away rotations
14. Will likely need extended time of supervision to watch for relapses in poor behavior

---

Example:

A resident, Isaiah, had been identified early for poor professionalism and there were several faculty members and chief residents who addressed this issue directly with him. Unfortunately he lacked insight and he had a reason to explain away each scenario. Six months into his residency, he met with a remediation specialist who reviewed his first evaluation with him which commented on professionalism problems. The resident dismissed the concern, giving an explanation. He was then presented with his second through sixth evaluations sequentially, all with the same comments. It wasn't until the sixth evaluation that he realized how he was being perceived and that they could not all be explained away.

A discussion ensued on the relevance of poor professionalism, as well as the academic and professional consequences. Even if he didn't truly believe that his behavior was unprofessional, he did understand the long-term consequences of being perceived as unprofessional and that was enough motivation to work on changing his behavior. I often say, "Despite your best intentions, this is how you are being perceived. Since you can't change others, how can you change so that the perception matches your intentions and you don't get in trouble?"

Behavior guidelines were set and examples were given and discussed as to how his prior behavior could have been better. Had he not agreed to work on his behavior, a mental health evaluation and letter of warning would have been warranted.

Isaiah's behavior continued to improve throughout residency, and he not only graduated at the top of his class but was readily hired by the university in which he did his residency.

In cases in which a learner appears to have no insight, I let her/him know that despite commendable motivation, s/he needs to change others' impression of her/his behavior. This is not done be changing others, but by empowering the learner to change how s/he presents herself/himself to others. Continue to emphasize the selfish reasons as to why s/he should be invested in the remediation process. Eventually, even though less than ideal, you will get buy-in on some level. Aristotle said, "We acquire virtues by having first put them into action... we become just by the practice of just actions, self-controlled by exercising self-control and courageous by performing acts of courage." Changing behavior can change one's beliefs about the need for professional behavior.

8. Step-by-Step Approach to the Remediation of Practice-Based Learning and Improvement

Practice-Based Learning and Improvement is identified much less frequently as one in which the learner is deficient and that may be due to the fact that it overlaps with other competencies or that evaluators are less familiar with the criteria for this competency. Without a doubt, insight and self-awareness and willingness to acknowledge one's deficits are key to the remediation of practice-based learning and improvement.

To role model this competency, I announce at the start of a rotation that the learners should expect regular feedback from me and that I will expect regular feedback from them. I also say, "If I ask you a question and you do not know the answer, then I expect you to look it up and report back the next day. Likewise, if you ask me a question and I do not know the answer, I will look it up and report back to you."

1. Meet with the Success Team to review the remediation plan, methods for learner reassessment and goals for successful remediation
    a. Program, course, or clerkship director
    b. Faculty interested in leading the remediation
    c. The learner
2. Ask the learner to explore and write about
    a. Her/his strengths and weaknesses
    b. The benefits of continued learning

    c. What s/he believes the current expectations are
    d. What s/he believes the lifelong expectations are
    e. The pros and cons of receiving feedback
    f. The importance of acknowledging one's own limitations and seeking help when needed
3. Review the above components of practice-based learning and improvement with the learner
    a. Include how the lack of independent learning and willingness to accept feedback is received by faculty and colleagues
    b. Discuss the need for setting new learning and patient care goals
4. Identify what you expect the learner to be doing and set a time frame
    a. Identifying one question to look up on each patient
    b. Reading nightly on patient cases to answer these questions
    c. Utilize scientific studies to modify practice
    d. Seeking feedback and trying different strategies based on feedback
5. To improve insight, consider having the learner do a quality improvement project for which s/he reviews her/his own charts. This will undoubtedly highlight concrete examples of the need for improvement
6. Model behavior
    a. Help the learner identify questions to look up
    b. Model appropriate verbal and action responses to receiving feedback and have the learner practice them
7. For assessment to measure progress consider
    a. Supervising faculty evaluations
    b. Written or clinical exam scores demonstrating progressive improvement

---

Example:

An intern, Maggie, was in a competition with her peers to see who could get in more days on the ski slopes that year. It became very clear that while very book smart upon admission, her colleagues were rapidly surpassing her at an exponential pace and she was falling behind. She was resistant to such feedback and had not been setting personal goals to improve her skills. I remember drawing her this graph, charting her performance relative to her peers. Note that ski season started in November.

While not in need of formal remediation, I pulled her aside and asked her to explore the importance of continued learning and what she believed the expectations to be. She knew exactly what to say and, therefore, also knew the

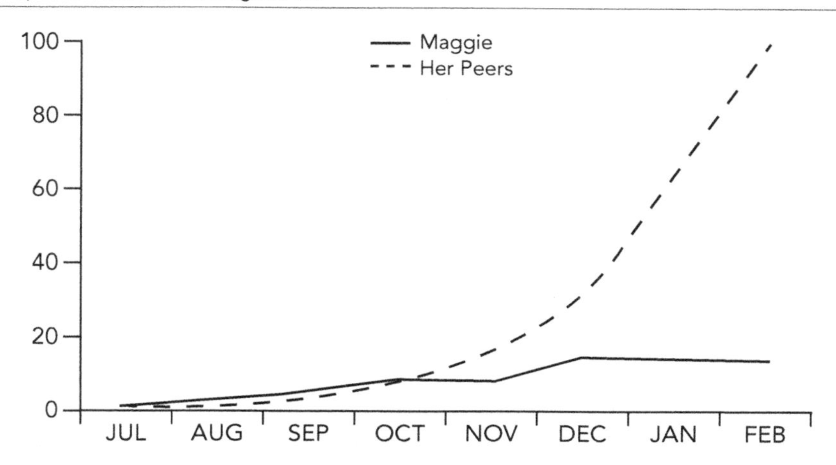

FIGURE 8.1 A Visual Description of the Struggling Learner's Progress Relative to Her Peers

educational expectations. She accepted the feedback politely, but I wondered if I had gotten through to her. Her performance was passable and she was not enrolled in the remediation program. At the end of training, Maggie failed her specialty board examination.

With this newly found insight and the benefit of hindsight, she is now on board with creating a plan for self-directed learning and wants to catch up on all of the opportunities for ongoing learning she has missed. Throughout the day, she started recording any question she wanted to look up in the evening. She dutifully read articles to answer her questions each night. Maggie spontaneously admitted, or rather confessed, regret as the process would have been much easier had she listened to the feedback and been committed to self directed learning years ago.

9. Step-by-Step Approach to the Remediation of Systems-Based Practice

The competency of systems-based practice overlaps with interpersonal skills and professionalism. As with Practice-Based Learning and Improvement, this competency is identified much less frequently and I suspect that it is for the same reasons. General faculty are often not exactly sure what this competency includes.

1. Meet with the Success Team to review the remediation plan, methods for learner reassessment and goals for successful remediation

   a. Program, course, or clerkship director
   b. Faculty interested in leading the remediation
   c. The learner
2. Ask the learner to explore the benefits of
   a. Interprofessional and multidisciplinary teamwork
   b. The value of multiple perspectives and input
   c. The complexity of the health care system for clinicians and patient
   d. Risk benefit analysis for patient care
   e. The future of medicine and stewardship of resources
3. Review the above components of systems-based practice as it relates to your geographic area
   a. What are the health care resources in your institution and local area?
   b. What patient care resources are available?
   c. How does insurance impact access to resources?
   d. Review key components of patient handoffs (aka handovers) and transitions of care
   e. How does one best advocate for her/his patients?
4. Identify the expectations and set a timeframe for achieving those expectations
   a. Expect to return patient phone calls within 24 hours
   b. Complete paperwork within 48 hours
   c. Send discharge summaries with patients
   d. Set up home health care services by the end of the day
   e. Lead the health care team and incorporate others' input to maximize patient care quality
5. For assessment to measure progress consider
   a. Supervising faculty evaluations and 360 degree evaluations

---

Example:

The chief resident, Ebenezer, did not value the multidisciplinary team meetings with the other residents, nurses, social workers and case managers. He refused to participate in the team meetings because he felt they were low yield and a waste of time. The remediation specialist, program director and Ebenezer sat down to discuss his behavior. Aside from reminding him that the multidisciplinary team meetings were mandatory, they explored ways of making the team meetings higher yield and how the chief could be a leader in improving these meetings. What could he ask of the attendees that would make the meetings more valuable for him and others at the meeting? If he helped maximize the productivity of the meetings, it would result in fewer pages and interruptions throughout the day for her/him, the nurses, social workers and case managers. The largest motivating factors for participation in the meetings seemed to be fewer interruptions, followed by being able to provide more consistent information and care to the patients. He was also asked to consider the perspectives of and impact of his behavior on the other attendees. Progress in this competency was monitored through 360 degree evaluations, through which he demonstrated more meaningful participation in the meetings.

10. Step-by-Step Approach to the Remediation of Mental Well-Being

And last, but certainly not least, is the competency entitled mental well-being. This is such a broad category that I have done my best to distill the algorithm down to the common overarching methods of approach.

1. Meet with the Success Team to review the remediation plan, methods for learner reassessment and goals for successful remediation
    a. Program, course or clerkship director
    b. Faculty interested in leading the remediation
    c. The learner
2. Discuss concerns about the learner's performance and concerns for the learner's well-being
3. Ask the learner to explore her/his concerns and yours
    a. Is this a new problem?
    b. Are there specific things preventing or limiting her/his performance?
    c. What has s/he done to improve her/his performance or to address obstacles?
    d. Has s/he ever been told that s/he has a learning disability or psychiatric illness? If so, discuss the treatment
    e. Does s/he use addictive substances on a weekly basis? Has s/he used illicit drugs or non-prescribed addictive pharmaceuticals since starting medical school?
4. Trust your instincts and clinical acumen more than what the learner reveals
    a. Know that when a learner struggles with substance abuse or other mental health issues that personal life is affected first (and work last)
    b. If either are affecting work, know that the problem has reached a critical level
    c. Do not neglect to ask the learner specifically about each of the following

        1. Psychosocial stressors
        2. Depression
        3. Anxiety
        4. Learning Disabilities or Difficulties
        5. Substance Use

5. Seek out local resources
    a. Mental health services based on the learner's insurance and resources available on campus
    b. Disabilities Office
    c. The Federation of State Physician Health Programs at www.fsphp.org to help address
        i. Substance use disorders
        ii. Mental Health
        iii. Behavioral Health
        iv. Stress
        v. Burnout
        vi. Physical Illness
        vii. Legal issues
6. If the learner is unwilling to participate in voluntary evaluation and treatment, require a mandatory psychiatric evaluation referral for learners with
    a. Inconsistent performance of unclear etiology
    b. Problems with attitude and/or motivation or suspected learning disabilities if not already documented through neuropsychiatric testing
        i. Consider neuropsychiatric testing if your learner in not making any progress, or appears to be "unteachable" despite good effort on the part of the learner
    c. Psychosocial stressors
    d. Suspected psychiatric diagnoses
    e. Substance abuse
7. All learners with this difficulty will need to have a supportive environment, fostered by faculty and the program director and/or remediation team
8. Activities to promote resident camaraderie may help significantly. Depending on the milieu, a learner support group may be beneficial, as well as organizations like Rachel Naomi Remen, MD's the "Healer's Art Courses" or "Finding Meaning in Medicine"
9. Since the problems within this category vary greatly, the remediation must be customized to the problem

   a. The mentor and learner together should establish specific goals for remediation and plan a remediation strategy
      i. Addressing the underlying cause
      ii. Discussing stress reduction techniques
      iii. Establishing tools and management skills to overcome the deficits while the etiology is being directly addressed
      iv. May require a leave of absence
         1. Issues to resolve, i.e., divorce, dying family member, bankruptcy
         2. Therapy and medications start to work, i.e. 4–6 weeks for antidepressants and attention deficit hyperactivity disorder medications
         3. Substance abuse treatment
10. Supportive feedback will be both constructive and encouraging
    a. Demonstrates to the learner your level of investment in her/his success
    b. Attachment to a mentor is often the most effective intervention
11. Watch for relapses in mental well-being from depression to anxiety to recurrent substance use.

Mandatory evaluations ***are*** necessary. These learners have severe enough problems to land them in remediation. There is no time to lose and their careers are at stake. The learner's well-being must be emphasized so that the referral is not viewed as punitive. Contact the Federation of State Physician Health Programs, www.fsphp.org, to determine the resources available in your state. Many states offer independent, confidential organizations, separate from state licensing boards that provide diagnostic evaluations and treatment referrals for physicians, including residents and medical students who have emotional, psychological or medical issues which, if left untreated could affect their ability to practice medicine. Through physician health programs and the equivalent for nurse practitioners, fitness for duty can also be professionally assessed and substance abuse testing obtained.

Example:

The clerkship director called both the director of the remediation program and the Student Affairs dean immediately on learning that a student, Carlos, had been missing for over 48 hours. The call was correctly made directly to the personal cell phones of each person to ensure rapid contact, regardless of the time of day or other events going on. The remediation specialist and dean spoke to each other and, given the learner's history, contacted the police to help find him and do a welfare check. This behavior was very much out of character. The primary goal was to ensure the student's safety. Carlos was found in a psychotic and manic state, driving erratically across county lines. He was brought to the hospital on a mental health hold for psychiatric evaluation and subsequent inpatient admission. He reported that his psychosis was related "to taking too many Ritalin (methylphenidate) and other prescribed medications." He was not permitted to return to work until a fitness for duty evaluation and a treatment plan arranged by the local Physicians' Health Program were completed. As always, PHP was extremely helpful in evaluating the student, determining fitness for duty and ensuring proper treatment and ongoing monitoring for Carlos.

He was able to return to class and graduated on time. He was monitored by a health program throughout residency and graduated at the top of his class, without another mental health crisis.

There are many examples of physicians with the range of Axis I psychiatric diagnoses that go on to have highly productive careers. I have seen first break learners with bipolar disorder and schizophrenia continue to practice and contribute greatly to our profession.

I often get questions about working with learners who have difficult personalities. Although it may be tempting, do not diagnose them. You are a clinician, but not the learner's clinician. Consider the following additional tips.

If the learner likes to be the center of attention, is vulnerable to the suggestions of others, has inappropriate seductive or provocative behavior and has overly exaggerated emotional expressions:

- Use direct language
- Use closed-ended questions for the learner rather than open-ended questions
- Teach the learner to speak with more detail, and ask for concrete examples
- Correct inconsistencies, especially if speech is exaggerated
- Give and enforce time limitations, such as for presentations
- Redirect the learner to keep her/him focused on the presenting problem
- If overly flirtatious, have a mentor of the same gender give her/him alternative ways of behaving and reinforce the ethics and conduct of the profession
- Be prepared to be politely persistent to affect change

If the learner is arrogant, manipulative, seeks admiration or has a grandiose sense of self-importance while lacking empathy for others:

- Provide brief amounts of dedicated undivided attention to the learner
- Enforce time limits, so that every member of the team gets the same amount of dedicated attention
- Acknowledge the value of her/his input as well as that of each individual on the team
- If possible, do not tell her/him that s/he is incorrect. Help lead her/him to the correct answer so s/he feels like s/he came up with it herself/himself or tell her/him what would be better or more correct

If the learner has recurrent difficulty working with others, impulsivity, has poorly controlled anger or is moody and divides others into those they idealize and those they don't respect:

- Don't take the learner's difficulties personally
- Do not try to undermine her/his already low self-esteem
- Discuss the learner's behaviors openly with the learner and, whenever possible, how it relates to professional conduct
- Redirect the learner back to relevant content for discussion
- Limit the number of people providing feedback to avoid splitting
- Work on expanding her/his understanding of concepts from black and white to shades of gray
- Provide structure and boundaries for establishing guidelines of behaviors and support her/his resilience in following the structure without giving in
- Give responsibility back to the learner and hold her/him accountable
- Limit the power given to the learner. Do not let her/him place herself/himself at the top of the hierarchy. It is up to you to create the rules or set the tone or culture

If the learner is shy, avoids activities, seems overly restrained or inhibited, socially detached and highly sensitive to criticism:

- Provide ample compliments and recognition of abilities and a supportive safety net when working through difficult cases
- Be mindful of making the learner feel valued and included and a necessary team player
- Encourage the learner to take a more active role and be more assertive for the sake of patient safety
- Give her/him opportunities to speak in safe environments

Don't forget

As a reminder, while I did not specifically highlight the 3 key steps for designing a remediation plan, if you go back and examine each algorithm you will see that each includes deliberate practice, feedback and self-assessment. All components are crucial to successful remediation and are the same components necessary to make average clinicians experts! (**Table 8.7**)

TABLE 8.7 Remediation Strategies for Each Deficit. The chart below highlights the key components associated with the remediation of each competency.

Deficit	Remediation Strategy
1. Medical Knowledge	• Learner should meet with remediation team • Identify knowledge goals and requirements of course • Identify how learner learns best • Assess the learner's level of knowledge; global or focal deficits • Review what the learner is reading—review material rather than primary articles • Emphasize learning why, rather than what or how • Change from disease based reading to symptom based reading • Create an ongoing list of items to look up • Link patient cases to reading • Give feedback and encourage self-reflection • Accommodations when necessary • Establish how s/he will be reassessed
2. Clinical Skills	• Learner should meet with remediation team • Identify skills gaps • Assign reading or videos on physical exam skills/procedures • Videotape student's performance of deficit skills • Review videotaped performance with student, addressing deficits and assessing self-awareness • Give feedback and demonstrate missed elements or errors

(continued)

TABLE 8.7 Remediation Strategies for Each Deficit (continued)

Deficit	Remediation Strategy
2. Clinical Skills (continued)	• Repetition and practice • Emphasize the use of clinical reasoning in performing clinical skills • Establish how s/he will be reassessed
3. Clinical Reasoning and Judgment	• Learner should meet with remediation team • Review new and old cases with the student • Create differential diagnosis (DDx) based on age, gender, chief complaint o include most likely, and what you don't want to miss • Provide a framework for clinical reasoning • Identify relevant HPI questions, PE elements, and ROS questions • Have you seen before or read about before? • Customize DDx and analyze each diagnosis: compare and contrast!! • Review diagnostic options o do nothing, order a lab, order a test, prescribe a medication • Review treatment options • Create an ongoing list of clinical questions to look up and apply to patient care • Teach student to use resources and residents/attendings for feedback • Chart stimulated recall with feedback • Have student reflect on consequences of choices • Establish how s/he will be reassessed
4. Time Management and Organization	• Learner should meet with remediation team • Review expectations • Obtain learner's perspective and concerns • Teach a data organization system • Model pre-rounding, have learner use same model with every patient • Identify tasks to be completed • Prioritize tasks • Identify length of time for each task • Have student keep a minute to minute log of daily activities • Give feedback

(continued)

TABLE 8.7 Remediation Strategies for Each Deficit (continued)

Deficit	Remediation Strategy
4. Time Management and Organization (continued)	• Have learner observe peers', residents' and others' strategies and discuss • May need lighter patient load • Stress management • Establish how s/he will be reassessed
5. Interpersonal Skills	• Learner should meet with remediation team • Review relevance of good interpersonal skills • Deficiencies or conflicts should be addressed directly and privately • Give specific examples of interpersonal conflicts • Have learner provide or model alternative examples of positive interaction in conflict • Self-reflection • View videotape for self-awareness • Consider mental health evaluation • Warning/Probation • Establish how s/he will be reassessed
6. Communication	• Learner should meet with remediation team • Review relevance of good communication • Have learner identify how communication throughout the workday can either facilitate or hinder patient care • Reading from communications textbook • Practice oral presentations emphasizing strong clinical reasoning • Practice summarizing complex cases • Practice specific skill sets, e.g., give bad news, interview about sensitive topic, ask questions, etc • View videotaped performance for self-awareness. If using standardized patients, give feedback and repeat • Consider Bayer Workshops • Role modeling—observe preceptor using Calgary-Cambridge Observation Guide • Teach learner to clarify communication throughout her/his day • Establish how s/he will be reassessed

(continued)

TABLE 8.7 Remediation Strategies for Each Deficit (continued)

Deficit	Remediation Strategy
7. Professionalism	• Learner should meet with remediation team • Review the relevance of being professional from your perspective and *her/his* (remind her/him of the consequences of being perceived as unprofessional!) • Set expectations • Review specific examples of her/his unprofessional behavior • Emphasize high level of accountability • Self-reflection • Official warning, probation and/or send to promotions committee • Limit setting • Establish how s/he will be reassessed
8. Practice-Based Learning and Improvement	• Learner should meet with remediation team • Ask the learner to identify her/his strengths and weaknesses • Ask the learner to explore and write about the benefits of continued learning • Clarify the expectations • Ask the learner to write a self-reflection piece that includes the purposes of feedback and independent learning and a reflection on the feedback s/he has received • Review how her/his responses are perceived • Discuss implementation of new knowledge from scientific studies and/or different strategies based on feedback • Have learner complete quality improvement projects that will shed light on her/his practice • Model appropriate responses to feedback and how to incorporate self-directed learning • Establish how s/he will be reassessed
9. Systems-Based Practice	• Learner should meet with remediation team • Ask the learner to explore the benefits of interprofessional input and team collaboration

(continued)

TABLE 8.7 Remediation Strategies for Each Deficit (continued)

Deficit	Remediation Strategy
9. Systems-Based Practice (continued)	• Help the learner improve patient care by seeking health care resources, understanding how the healthcare system impacts care and the value of transitions of care • Teach the learner to advocate for his patients • Set expectations with a timeframe for meeting expectations • Establish how s/he will be reassessed
10. Mental Well-Being	• Learner should meet with remediation team • Discuss concerns with student and her/his reflections • Refer for psychiatric evaluation for learning disabilities, psychiatric diagnosis, and substance abuse (www.fsphp.org) o assess for fitness for duty, evaluation and treatment • Provide supportive environment and schedule • Teams and activities that promote camaraderie • Stress reduction • Skills to overcome deficits • Feedback • Establish how s/he will be reassessed

CHAPTER 9:

Determining Success of Remediation and Reassessment

How should we judge "success or failure"? What is success? Is success seeing a learner through to the completion of her/his academic program, mentoring a learner towards an area of medicine more suited to their skills and/or encouraging an unsafe or unmotivated learner to find a new career? These are all examples of success in my mind, if you, as a teacher, have given remediation a fair, honest and valiant effort.

Fortunately, most learners go on to succeed within their academic programs. Two criteria can be used to determine the success of remediation of a given deficit.

1. Has the resident shown significant improvement *and* caught up to her/ his level of training in the previously deficient competency(ies)?
2. Is the improvement sustainable?

Following remediation, the learner must be formally assessed for the criteria above. Often the faculty members directly involved in remediation are asked to provide the assessment, because they are so dedicated and available; however, this is a conflict of interest. The remediation faculty member is biased in that he wants the learner to demonstrate improvement for the learner's sake, her/his own emotional investment in the learner and also her/his own personal success as a remediation specialist.

Reassessment *must* whenever possible be performed by a blinded and neutral party. Most of the deficits are not content specific. If you have a small residency program, consider having a faculty member from another specialty conduct the reassessment. For example, if an orthopedic surgery resident is struggling with communication skills or organization, an internal medicine, family medicine physician, or general surgeon can provide the reassessment.

Reassessment can be done using any of the following assessment methods:

- Repeat the clinical block, or portion of the block with a new team
- Standardized patient encounters

- Objective structured clinical examinations
- Mini-clinical evaluation examinations
- Brief structured clinical examinations
- Simulation
- Directly observed encounters with actual patients
- Clinical evaluation exercises
- Multiple choice exams
- Written or web-based assessments
- Chart reviews and chart-stimulated recall
- Supervisor or peer observations
- Multi-source evaluations
- Patient and procedure logs
- Critique of journal articles
- Responses to self-assessment

Specific reassessment tools were recommended with the algorithms in Chapter 8 and may vary based on resources, timing and faculty availability (also see **Table 9.1**).

TABLE 9.1 Reassessment Options Based on Deficit

Competency	Reassessment Options
1. Medical Knowledge	• Written or web-based knowledge assessments • Multiple choice exams
2. Clinical Skills	• Objective structured clinical examinations (OSCE) or Standardized patient encounters • Simulation • Repeating part or all of a rotation • Procedure logs
3. Clinical Reasoning and Judgment	• Written or web-based case-based assessments • Standardized patient encounters or OSCE • Mini-clinical evaluation examinations • Chart-stimulated recall • Repeating part or all of a rotation

(continued)

TABLE 9.1 Reassessment Options Based on Deficit (continued)

Competency	Reassessment Options
4. Time Management and Organization	• Direct observation • Repeating part or all of a rotation • Multi-source evaluations • Patient and procedure logs
5. Interpersonal Skills	• Direct observation • Standardized patient encounters or OSCE • Mini-clinical evaluation examinations • Multi-source evaluations • Responses to self-reflection
6. Communication	• Direct observation • Standardized patient encounters or OSCE • Mini-clinical evaluation examinations • Multi-source evaluations
7. Professionalism	• Direct observation • Multi-source evaluations • Responses to self-reflection • Patient and procedure logs
8. Practice-Based Learning and Improvement	• Responses to self-reflection • Evaluation from supervisors • Critique of journal articles
9. Systems-Based Practice	• Direct observation • Multi-source evaluations
10. Mental Well-being	• Direct observation • Evaluations from supervisors • Repeat part or all of a rotation • Psychiatric evaluation, fitness for duty

This has been a long dense set of chapters, full of lists. Let's take time to review this section with a few cases.

CHAPTER 10:

Remediation Cases

The cases provided in Section 1 Chapter 4 were written based on real cases, with identifying information removed. You will be asked to revisit these cases and develop a remediation strategy.

If you had any difficulty completing the outline below, revisit the step-by-step approaches to remediation in chapter 8.

Case 1

Please review Case #1 from Chapter 4 and fill in the blanks. Your task is to create a remediation strategy based on the SINGLE greatest deficit.

Which deficit are you targeting?

____

What would you have this learner practice?

____

____

____

____

____

____

How would you structure feedback for this learner?

____

____

____

On what should this learner reflect?

____

____

CASE 1: REFLECTION

The remediation of this learner required a 3-month intervention. It involved the clerkship director, a faculty member who specialized in remediation, an additional inpatient attending and working with a resident team on a general medicine ward service. Wilbur's clinical reasoning was significantly behind his peers and he was unable to make substantial progress while on clinical rotations.

He was relieved of his clinical responsibilities for 3 weeks. During this time, Wilbur met with the remediation specialist 3 times a week for 1–2 hours per session to review cases as per the algorithm described for the remediation of clinical reasoning and judgment.

Following the intervention, he was placed on a rotation with a blinded team, who did not know of his previous deficits. The student was encouraged to let the team know that he wanted to work on clinical reasoning during this rotation and he did so. He successfully completed the sub-internship and graduated from medical school.

CASE 2:

Please review Case #2 from Chapter 4 and fill in the blanks. Your task is to create a remediation strategy based on the SINGLE greatest deficit.

Which deficit are you targeting?

___

What would you have this learner practice?

___

___

___

___

___

___

How would you structure feedback for this learner?

___

___

___

On what should this learner reflect?

___

___

CASE 2: REFLECTIONS

The remediation of this learner required a 1-month intervention. It involved a faculty member specializing in communication, the remediation specialist and standardized patients. Jane had struggled with communication her entire life, had insight and was very invested in the remediation process.

Jane was removed from her clinical rotations for 3 afternoons to work with the standardized patients. In addition to following the algorithm for remediation, I would like to outline a few specifics. During this time, she was asked to interact with the standardized patients as if they were real patients, completing a thorough history and physical and multiple focused interviews on medical and social complaints. The 2 faculty members, via video from another room, viewed her performance live. At the completion of each case, the standardized patient gave Jane feedback as did each of the faculty members. She was given specific instruction on her strengths and weaknesses and then given a concrete plan to improve her weaknesses with the next encounter.

Example:

"Instead of asking a series of questions, respond to what the patient tells you. If at the end of the interview, you did not get enough information, then ask specific direct questions to collect that information."

Jane's progress was remarkable from case to case. She appeared to have no difficulty incorporating the feedback. She was a highly intelligent and motivated individual who just needed more direction and guidance than her peers.

Following the intervention, her progress was monitored on subsequent clinical rotations and she continued to demonstrate improvement in her communication skills, scored well on her evaluations in all competencies including communications and passed all of her rotations. She graduated on time and matched into a very competitive specialty and residency program.

Case 3:

Please review Case #3 from Chapter 4 and fill in the blanks. Your task is to create a remediation strategy based on the SINGLE greatest deficit.

Which deficit are you targeting?

____

What would you have this learner practice?

____

____

____

____

____

____

How would you structure feedback for this learner?

____

____

____

On what should this learner reflect?

____

____

CASE 3: REFLECTIONS

The remediation of this learner required a 6-month intervention. It involved the program director, the remediation specialist, and chief resident. Dr. Lo struggled with interpersonal skills, which was further complicated by the fact that she was from another culture and English was her second language.

Dr. Lo went through the remediation plan outlined in the approach to the remediation of interpersonal skills. She met weekly with the remediation specialists to explore alternative interpersonal styles and options. It took 6–8 weeks for the learner to acknowledge that the problem was hers and not attributed to others. It was not until then that she was able to make any meaningful progress. We discussed verbal language, body language, perceived attitude and intentions. She explored how to communicate the same information and ask the same questions in an acceptable manner, considering both the intended and unintended audiences. She explored team dynamics, the hierarchy of medicine and how to value all members of the team.

Dr. Lo was given a letter of warning and had moonlighting and away rotations restricted. Her progress had its ups and downs, but overall she demonstrated improvement. Since the chief resident was frequently receiving unsolicited feedback on Dr. Lo's interactions from other residents, students, nurses and attendings, the chief was in the best position to monitor Dr. Lo's progress and notify the remediation specialist when a new conflict arose. Her evaluations were also monitored for improvement. With firm requirements that she was to uphold the behavior guidelines, she graduated on time and matched into the subspecialty of her choice.

Self-Assessment Quiz for Section 2

1. A resident comes to you unsolicited to report that his medical student is struggling. You should do which of the following (check all that apply)
   a. Discuss the resident's concerns and ask for examples
   b. Ask the resident to send you a brief email regarding his concerns
   c. Investigate the concerns to determine if this is a trend that needs intervention, if this is an isolated serious problem that needs intervention or if this is something to monitor closely
   d. Make sure the learner received direct feedback regarding the concerns
   e. Consider reporting the concerns on the student's evaluation
2. Further investigation reveals that this student arrives too late to complete his morning work, is frequently disorganized in appearance and forgets to wear his white coat. It appears that the student is struggling with time management and organization, professionalism and mental well-being. Discussions with the student reveal that he ran out of his ADHD medication and has not been able to make a follow-up appointment to get a prescription since starting third year. He is afraid that asking for time off will make him look bad. Which deficit(s) do you want to address in your remediation plan?
   a. Time management and organization
   b. Professionalism
   c. Mental well-being
   d. All of the above
3. The remediation plan should include
   a. Deliberate practice
   b. Feedback
   c. Self-reflection
   d. All of the above
4. At the completion of remediation, the student must
   a. Have his skills reassessed by the faculty doing remediation and the progress documented in the student's evaluation
   b. Have his skills reassessed by an independent faculty member and the progress documented in the student's evaluation
   c. Know that the next block director will be notified of the concerns and that his progress will be documented in his evaluation
   d. Assume remediation was successful and never look back

5. How should we judge "success or failure"?
   a. The student has shown significant improvement
   b. The student's performance has caught up to his or her level of training
   c. Performance is sustained during remediation

Section 2 Self-Assessment Answers

1. All of the choices should be addressed.
2. (c) Encourage the student to make a doctor's appointment and relieve him of his clinical responsibilities without penalty, so that he may go to that appointment. If the student does not have a provider, a list can often be obtained from the Student Affairs Office.
3. (d) All of the above.
4. (b) Reassessment should be performed by a blinded and neutral party and it should be noted on the student's evaluation in comments, so that the student's progress can be followed longitudinally by a process independent of grades. At this time, notifying the subsequent block director is discouraged; however, you can empower the student to guide his education by focusing on his weaknesses (i.e., during this rotation, I would like to work on improving my presentations).
5. (b) While improvement is encouraging, the deficit must be corrected to the expectations for his level of training. True sustainability needs to be measured after the supports of a remediation plan are gone.

SECTION 3:

Giving Feedback to the Struggling Learner

Failing finals is often a surprise for the student but not the teacher.

J Cleland, R Arnold, A Chessar*

*From Cleland, Jennifer, Rachelle Arnold, and Alistair Chesser. "Failing finals is often a surprise for the student but not the teacher: identifying difficulties and supporting students with academic difficulties." *Medical teacher* 27.6 (2005): 504–508.

CHAPTER 11:

Key Elements of Giving Difficult Feedback

Oksana is a 2nd year emergency medicine resident. Prior to signing out Mr. Chen to the next shift's resident, she performed a lumbar puncture. Despite having ordered a PT/INR, she failed to check it prior to the procedure. The INR was 9. He went on to have bleeding into the spinal canal with devastating effects. Oksana needs to receive feedback on this devastating oversight. Unfortunately, it is not her first mistake. You are unable to sleep all night in anticipation of what will be a very difficult conversation tomorrow morning.

If you give brief feedback to your learners every day and periodic formal feedback, have you seen improvement in all of your learners? Are you completely comfortable giving negative or constructive feedback? I have been working in this area extensively for years and still feel the need for more resources and more opportunities for self-awareness and insight. Here are some of my favorite studies on remediation.

1. Holmboe et al. conducted a prospective observational study on feedback sessions following a mini-clinical evaluation exercise (mini CEX). Without specific prior instruction on how to give feedback, faculty were instructed to engage the learner in a feedback session. Despite this, only 80% actually gave feedback. Of the feedback given, 61% pertained to learner reaction, 34% requested self-assessment and only 8% involved an action plan. He concluded that specific instruction is needed if we want our faculty to include the key elements of meaningful feedback. Even when asked to give feedback in the setting of being watched, few faculty members gave effective feedback. An action plan was given to only 1 in 12 students, leaving the rest potentially vulnerable to failure.
2. Hodges et al. conducted a study in which residents rated their performance in breaking bad news to a standardized patient. The study illustrated that residents in the bottom third of the class overestimated their own abilities, while residents in the top third of the class underestimated their abilities. All residents

regardless of ability felt that their performance was average. Learners need our feedback to get an accurate representation of their abilities.

3. ML Boehler conducted a randomized control trial of medical students' reactions to feedback. Two groups were given the same instructions on how to make 2-handed surgical knots. The students were then randomized to receive either specific feedback or general compliments. Their performance was videotaped and assessed, as was the students' satisfaction. In short, specific feedback improved performance on procedural skills; however, students were less satisfied. So I tell my learners about this study and then say, "I can either give you feedback that will make you feel good or I can give you feedback that will make you a better clinician, and my job is to make you a better clinician."

According to the American Board of Internal Medicine, feedback is a "process by which the teacher provides learners with information about their performance for the purposes of improving their performance." Working with struggling learners is a challenge and at times you will get frustrated. Be sure that all of your feedback is given with the goal of making the learner a better clinician. Resist using it as a conscious or unconscious opportunity to vent your frustrations.

We all have different communication styles and it will be important for you to learn how to use your style most effectively. What types of conversations are you most skilled at having? Are you subconsciously more willing to have these conversations and therefore do so more often? What about the conversations that you fear? Think of ways that you have avoided these conversations in the past. How can you improve on this in the future? Perhaps you have a colleague who is better at giving difficult feedback. Invite them to join your feedback session, watch them, model their behavior and get input on your feedback from your colleagues and the learners themselves. Sometimes you may want an additional person in the room as a witness or mediator, depending on the volatility of the learner or perceived potential legal risks of the encounter.

Now, let's review the key elements of giving effective feedback (followed by a summary in **Table 11.1**).

Key Elements of Meaningful Feedback

SET EXPECTATIONS: Giving effective feedback requires content, location, timing, and technique; however, the *first step is always to set expectations* for your learners upfront. Feedback is most successful when the expectations are

TABLE 11.1 Tips on Giving Feedback

- Decide on brief or formal feedback
- Identify observable behaviors to commend and behaviors to correct
- Limit to 2 or 3 areas
- Choose the location—private or public
- Identify optimal timing
- Label it "Feedback"
- Be unequivocally clear
- Summarize the feedback
- Commit to a plan
- Repeat feedback on the same issues later in the rotation
- Elicit input on your feedback

verbalized at the beginning of the rotation. Ideally, there will be stated goals and objectives for each rotation, to which you can add your personal expectations based on your style of teaching.

Example:

Jing, you should have received the goals and objectives for this rotation. Let's review those together. Also, I would like to add 2 expectations. Calculate creatinine clearance on all of your patients and please complete all necessary calculations prior to rounds, such as those of anion gaps, fractional excretions of sodium and creatinine clearance.

CONTENT: The next step in giving feedback is observation. It begins the very first moment you meet your learner and start working together. Physicians have well developed clinical observation skills that can be used to assess their learners' abilities. In preparation for giving feedback, take a moment to reflect on your learner's performance. Consider the learner's abilities and performance in each of the ACGME Competencies "Plus." Identify the learner's strengths and weaknesses. This will help prepare you to give both reinforcing and corrective feedback. Try to use firsthand experiences you have witnessed as opposed to second hand information.

Choose 2–3 content areas to focus your constructive feedback and make sure that the areas relate to the learner's actions and behaviors and not to her/him personally. Feedback should present information rather than judgment. So that there is no confusion or misunderstanding, choose content that is specific and unequivocally clear.

Example:

"Renata, my feedback for you today is to work on organizing the patient's assessment and plan. Start by prioritizing the problem list with the most important problem first and the least active problem last. Within each problem state the differential diagnosis, followed by your analysis of the diagnoses, then diagnostic work-up and lastly the treatment plan."

As faculty, we must be conscious of our non-verbal feedback as it may give unintended false confidence.

Example:

Nodding your head to hurry a slow presenter along may be seen as encouragement that s/he is doing a good job and should keep going.

LOCATION AND LEARNING ENVIRONMENT: Once you have determined the content of your feedback, you can consider both time and place. Try to give feedback as soon as possible. If the learner is angry, overwhelmed or hurried, find a better time to give feedback as s/he may be too distracted to listen and learn from what you have to say. Relocating may be necessary to give negative feedback privately, unless you believe it is feedback that would benefit your team and everyone else in earshot. Perhaps you wish to commend your learner where s/he can be appropriately recognized and you want to choose a more public place, like on rounds. If you have one stellar learner and one weaker learner, be careful not to overemphasize that difference by always giving positive feedback to the stronger one in front of the weaker one.

Example:

You are in a private conference room with your residents and students. After noting that the learning environment is safe, you say, "Joe, I'd like to give you some feedback on the presentation you just gave the team. Your presentations today were very clear and easy to follow, and contained all of the pertinent data; however, you like your peers, need to be sure to present at least 3 differential diagnoses for each active problem."

TIMING: Effective feedback requires a multifaceted approach utilizing both brief daily doses and less frequent, but more detailed formal sessions.

The former provides the learner with short (1–3 minutes) feedback with each interaction.

Example:

"Sarah, your history of present illness was very concise and you chose the most pertinent review of systems questions to include."

Example:

"Adam, you did a great job incorporating and inviting feedback from everyone at the multidisciplinary meeting today."

Example:

"Jean, you communicated very well with Mr. Smith and his family yesterday during that challenging palliative care meeting. You listened well and really did a great job addressing their concerns."

The latter utilizes a more formal (5–20 minutes) structure and commonly occurs at both the middle and end of the rotation. This gives you time to address all pertinent areas of performance. Be sure to summarize the formative feedback at the end of the session and establish a plan for moving forward. Feedback alone does not change or improve performance. It is the plans and goals that learners set in response to feedback that lead to change. Have your learner write down the plan and make a commitment to move forward with her/his education through feedback. If feedback is given early enough in your interaction, it will allow the learner to implement the plan and demonstrate improvement within the same clinical setting.

TECHNIQUES: When you begin giving feedback, be sure to let the learner know that you are going to give her/him feedback. Be sure to use the actual word "feedback" because if it is not labeled, the learner may not remember that you gave them feedback. As one of my mentors says, "I'm giving you permission to use the F-word."

There are many styles in the approach to giving feedback. While they are more commonly employed during formal feedback sessions they can also be employed during brief feedback sessions. Some use the "sandwich model" where the learner is given positive, then negative, and then positive feedback, followed by an action plan. An alternate method is to "ask, tell, ask." In this model, the interaction starts by asking the learner to reflect on her/his performance. Usually, this takes the pressure off the person giving feedback, because most learners are harder on themselves than the person offering feedback. You may also quickly learn that your learner lacks insight and that is also helpful. Then, the faculty member gives the learner both reinforcing and corrective feedback and asks the learner about her/his understanding of the feedback and guides her/him in developing the plan. Additionally, a hybrid model is also effective. It starts with reflection first, followed by positive, negative, positive feedback, and then the creation of a plan.

When giving feedback, remember to be specific, identify what was done well and what was not done well (see **Table 11.2**). Depersonalize the critique by clearly addressing her/his work and not her/him personally. Focus on your perceptions of her/his work and encourage self-reflection. Don't forget to end with a plan for moving forward! Let the learner know that you will be monitoring her/him to see that s/he has implemented the plan and that you will provide feedback as s/he makes progress.

Feedback is not easy, especially when your learner is struggling. It gets easier with practice and eventually becomes second nature, even when giving difficult feedback. Be honest with your learner and with yourself. If you are professional and respectful in giving feedback and the learner understands that you have her/his best interest in mind, s/he will eventually realize that you are not against her/him, but rather working towards the same goal.

While many of the key tenets of providing feedback apply to all levels of learners, there are some unique differences in giving effective feedback to struggling learners. *Struggling learners, unlike the higher achievers, benefit from feedback that is more immediate, directive and provides a framework.*

After giving formal or constructive feedback, be sure to follow-up with an email summarizing your discussion, concerns and steps for moving forward. People under stress don't always hear or remember and the email also provides legal documentation.

Establishing a culture of improvement requires a commitment to professional growth for both us as teachers and as learners and for our trainees. The most powerful way to change the current culture may be as simple a concept or as complicated a process as role modeling this change. Role model how to give and accept feedback, how to complete and receive an evaluation and how to create a plan to move forward to remediate one's own deficits. If you are open to accepting constructive criticism from your trainees, they will be much more receptive to yours. If you are willing to create a plan to remediate your deficits, your trainees will also be willing—and you will all become better physicians.

TABLE 11.2 How to Give Better Feedback

Unproductive Feedback	Moving Forward Through Feedback	Differences
Good job!	Good job in clearly identifying a question for the consultant.	Identifies what was done well.
You're great.	You are always reliable in following up on patient related tasks.	Refers to her/his work, rather than to her/him personally.
Your differential diagnosis is inadequate.	The differential diagnosis did not include pulmonary as well as cardiac causes of shortness of breath.	Specific, rather than general; implies expectations.
I hear that you are always leaving late.	I noticed that you had difficulty prioritizing your list of tasks today and had to stay late to complete them.	Firsthand data helps identify underlying issues.
The patient does not have iron deficiency anemia.	The patient has a different type of anemia. Let's look at the MCV: it shows a macrocytosis, which has other causes.	Corrects the reasoning as well as the answer.
You have no insight into your deficiencies.	I feel that you were uncomfortable giving bad news to the patient's family. Pay attention to this next time and let me know how you feel after the next encounter.	Your perception rather than judgment; encourages self-reflection.
You are rude and unprofessional.	It sounded like you were telling the nurse how to do her job. She will likely be more responsive if you talk about how you can work together to help your patient.	Your reflection is on the learner's behavior rather than on personality, also suggests a plan.

Self-Assessment Quiz for Section 3

1. Your learner has poor medical knowledge. You should:
   a. Compliment how intelligent the other members of the team are
   b. Tell your learner that s/he should read more
   c. Demonstrate that her/his knowledge is poor by pumping her/him on rounds
   d. State the topics or content areas that your learner should know
2. Corrective feedback is ineffective if it does not include:
   a. A private location
   b. A twenty minute discussion
   c. An action plan
   d. 3 examples
3. Which of the following is/are true?
   a. Giving feedback never gets any easier
   b. A collaborative versus antagonistic approach is the goal
   c. Faculty who give feedback have lower student ratings
   d. If a learner has a personality disorder, then it is helpful to discuss her/his personality rather than her/his behaviors

Section 3 Self-Assessment Answers

1. (d) Choice (d) sets the expectations and is specific. Choices (a) and (c) are divisive for the team and for your working relationship as teacher and student. Choice (b) is too vague and not specific enough.
2. (c) You must include an action plan. Learners often don't take the time to think through an action plan and, when they try, they have difficulty coming up with a plan of action.
3. (b) You should both be working towards the same goal. Giving feedback does get easier with practice. And, in case you are concerned, faculty who give feedback actually have higher student ratings. Lastly, stick to the rules—even when you have a most challenging learner.

SECTION 4:

Building a Remediation Program and Outcomes Data

Millions saw the apple fall, but Newton was the one who asked why.

Bernard Baruch[1]

Develop success from failures. Discouragement and failure are two of the surest stepping stones to success.

Dale Carnegie[2]

[1]From Bernard Baruch *New York Post* June 24, 1965.
[2]From Wilson, B. Sc Andrew. *The Price: The Education of a Fast-Oxidizer.* Author House, 2009.

CHAPTER 12:

Building a Remediation Program from the Ground Up

A remediation program must have at least the following components:

- A system of identification
- A remediation team for diagnosing the area(s) of deficiency and the development of a remediation plan
- Faculty development on how to access services for underperforming learners
- Measurable outcomes to determine success
- Financial resources and institutional backing
- Established policies and procedures

Remedial programs are most effective when they are centralized, are routinely evaluated, have a clearly defined philosophy, goals and objectives, integrate book learning with practical application and when there is institution wide commitment to remedial education.

A system for identification

In order to build a remediation program, you will have to establish thresholds by which learners are brought to the attention of the remediation team. These thresholds need to be standardized to ensure that they capture all struggling learners and that all learners are treated fairly and consistently. This helps ensure that struggling learners will not fall through the cracks.

In **Table 12.1**, suggested thresholds for identification are listed for each individual competency. This table omits 2 universal thresholds that are also included in our remediation program. First, the students should always be given the option of self-referral. Second, a course failure implies at least one deficit requiring remediation. The universal thresholds and the competency-based thresholds provide a redundant safety net for identifying underachieving learners. Depending on the competency and your training program, consider the following thresholds.

TABLE 12.1 Sample Threshold Measures for Determining Need for Remediation

Competency	Threshold for Identification
1. Medical Knowledge	Multiple choice question test score <75% or below 2 standard deviations of the mean
2. Clinical Skills	Clinical exam or simulation scores <70% or below 2 standard deviations of the mean OR An evaluation with a rating below 2 OR Comment indicating poor skills OR Procedural error OR Sparse procedure logs
3. Clinical Reasoning and Judgment	Clinical exam scores <70% or below 2 standard deviations of the mean OR An evaluation with a rating below 2 OR Comment indicating poor clinical reasoning and judgment OR Clinical incident
4. Time Management and Organization	Violating work hours OR Not completing work on time OR An evaluation with a rating below 2 OR Comment indicating poor time management and/or organization
5. Interpersonal Skills	2 or more reported conflicts OR An evaluation with a rating below 2 OR Comment indicating poor skills
6. Communication	Clinical exam scores <70% or below 2 standard deviations of the mean OR An evaluation with a rating below 2 OR Comment indicating poor communication

(continued)

TABLE 12.1 Sample Threshold Measures for Determining Need for Remediation (continued)

Competency	Threshold for Identification
7. Professionalism	>2 unexcused absences OR Arriving >10 minutes late >2 times OR Leaving early >3 times OR >2 reports of unprofessional behavior in any one course OR Incomplete assignment/requirements OR Reports in more than one course OR An egregious act of unprofessional behavior or illegal action, i.e. assault, falsification of records, sexual harassment
8. Practice-Based Learning and Improvement	Patient safety concern, not seeking help when needed OR An evaluation with a rating below 2 OR Multiple comments indicating resistance to feedback OR Multiple comments indicating lack of independent learning
9. Systems-Based Practice	An evaluation with a rating below 2 OR Comment indicating poor communication
10. Mental Well-being	Inconsistent Performance OR Not demonstrating improvement/not teachable OR Mental health impairing work performance

The most recent addition to the University of Colorado School of Medicine's institution-wide evaluation forms is a specific yes/no question that asks whether the learner needs remediation. The question is followed by an open comment box and the contact information for the remediation specialist, in case the evaluator wishes not to write additional comments. A "yes" to this question also meets the threshold for accessing remediation services. There was some debate as to whether this notification should be included in the evaluation and therefore seen by the learner. A decision was made to allow the learner to see the response to the question regarding the need for remediation, given the importance of feedback and letting the learner know how s/he is performing relative to expectations. For students specifically, this response does appear on their evaluation but not in their Medical Student Performance Evaluation or MSPE (aka Dean's letter). The decision to exclude this from the MSPE is to convey to the student that this is not punitive but a genuine request for additional information to maximize the student's potential. These students have enough red flags in their residency applications that their responses to this specific question are not needed to convey that they have struggled during training.

A remediation team for assistance with diagnoses and development of a remediation plan

Once a struggling learner is identified, there needs to be a clear policy and procedure for the development of a remediation plan.

Let's take a look at the flow sheet adapted from a chart originally created by Maureen Garrity, PhD at the University of Colorado School of Medicine (**Figure 12.1**).

Once a student is identified by meeting a threshold of poor performance, is self-referred, has a course failure or is referred by the course director, a social worker in the Student Affairs Office triages the concerns. If the student is having test taking problems, test taking anxiety, struggling with a learning disability, general communication difficulties or exhibits a mental health issue, s/he is referred to the non-clinician remediation specialist. The Department of Student Affairs can refer students to a social worker, psychiatrist, communication specialist or learning specialist. If the student is having an isolated clinical difficulty, such as difficulty writing a SOAP note, the learner may be referred directly to the clinical remediation specialist. The remediation specialist and learner would then come up with a plan for remediation of the deficit.

If the diagnosis is elusive or the remediation plan requires a more complicated approach with content-specific faculty, the need for additional resources or a

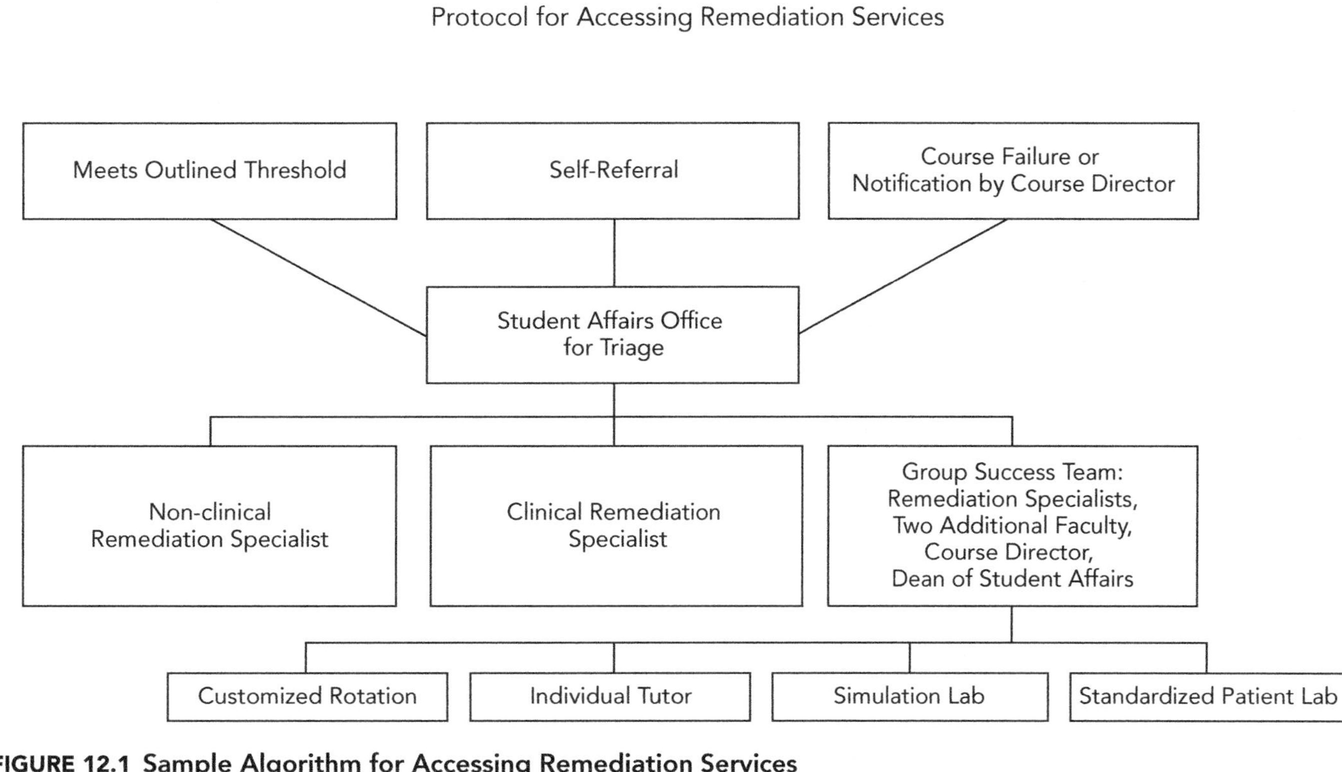

FIGURE 12.1 Sample Algorithm for Accessing Remediation Services

change to rotation or assignment schedules, a "Success Team" convenes with the learner. This team is comprised of 4–5 members, based on the needs of the learner, and the learner herself/himself. One of the team members is usually a psychiatrist. Together they come up with a plan for remediation of the ONE greatest deficit.

The benefits of convening a Success Team are that this group has the ability to customize rotation schedules, accommodate leaves of absence, provide individual tutoring and find funding for resources (if necessary) like the simulation lab or standardized patient lab. Of note, the promotions committee is an entity separate from Student Affairs and the remediation program, as the goal of the program is to capture struggling learners before they fail.

A similar model translates to residency and fellowship programs. Instead of notifying the Student Affairs Office, the program director is notified and the Success Team is the Resident Review Committee. The Resident Review Committee is made up of the chief residents, the program director, associate and assistant program directors, the remediation specialist and hospital site directors. As a committee, they determine the remediation resources and needs for letters of warning or for probationary status. The learner is notified by the program director and remediation specialist of the decisions of the committee in a written letter that outlines the following:

- Change in academic status from good to warning or probation
- The specific problematic performance with dates
- The ACGME competency related to the deficiency/problematic performance
- Goals of remediation
- Remediation plan
- If a mental health evaluation is required (this includes substance abuse testing)
- Measurable outcomes for success
- A time frame to demonstrate improvement, often 3 months
- Any restrictions, such as away rotations, electives, moonlighting, etc.
- The potential outcomes
    - Return to good standing
    - Continued warning or advanced to probation
    - Delays in training, suspension or termination if the learner fails to meet the conditions of the letter, or is an imminent risk to patients, self or others.

Notice that most decisions are made by group consensus, especially if the learner's status is changed from good academic standing to warning or probation, the learner's schedule is changed, or if the decision will be in any way reflected in her/his transcript or permanent record. Committee decisions protect organizations legally and individuals personally, sharing the responsibility for the decisions. This way no individual can be targeted as obstructing the learner's career.

Learners are permitted to rebut the concerns in writing or verbally. ACGME now requires appeal of all adverse actions. When it comes to deciding changes in academic status, grades or promotions, the remediation specialists act ONLY as the learner's advocate and do not participate in these decisions.

A team of faculty dedicated to remediation

The remediation program needs a director who will serve to build the program, propose written institutional policies and procedures, review and understand the institution's technical standards, monitor and modify the program based on results and feedback, provide faculty development and assist with remediation of learners. This is not a small task at any institution and 20–50% FTE funding would be required to do this job well.

In order to build a remediation program, a written proposal should be submitted to the Dean of the School of Medicine or Advanced Nurse Practice Program, the Designated Institutional Official or Director of Graduate Medical Education or leaders in similar high leadership positions. The proposal should include a recommended system of remediation, its importance to the institution and individual learners, the number of learners who will benefit from the program and the staffing and financial resources that will be required to build and then support the program.

Once the proposal is accepted, then policies and procedures can be written to build the program into your educational model. Development of a remediation program must include written policies and procedures to support the learner, the academic mission of the institution and the faculty leadership. First, decide who is responsible for remediation and reassessment. Is it the program or school, or the site or rotation where the deficit was detected? Without dedication and buy-in, I would caution you against the latter as it may detract from identification of struggling learners. Consider including the competency-specific expectations for each level of learner. Use your institution's technical standards to help guide your policies and procedures and to ensure equal treatment of all learners, including those with disabilities. Also include how a learner will be systematically identified for remediation, where documentation about the learner's remediation will be housed and who will have access to information about the learner. Describe the job functions of the remediation team members, and identify resources such as mental health professionals, learning disability specialists and legal advisors. Include who (not the remediation team) will measure learner success and the consequences for success and failure in meeting the measurable outcomes.

Be sure to include the degree of confidentiality or transparency of the information collected by the team. I stress transparency over confidentiality, so the learner knows who is aware of her/his struggles, what has been communicated and what the plan is. I am not a confidential advisor and do not promise confidentiality; however, I often keep details private and only disclose and convey the larger picture. For example, if a resident is going through a divorce, I would convey that the resident has a time limited personal stressor. You will want to address how the team is connected to the promotions committee and whether information about the learner will be revealed to subsequent course or rotation directors and/or evaluating faculty. My policy is to notify evaluating faculty only if there is a patient safety concern. If there is not a direct patient safety concern, I empower the learner to let her/his team know what her/his own personal learning objectives are for the rotation.

Lastly, be sure to outline the consequences of successful and failed remediation, such as delayed graduation, additional costs, probation or termination (see **Table 12.2**).

The program outcomes can be monitored based on learner outcomes via test scores, course grades, graduation rates, successful entry into the next level of training or career and completion or assimilation into this next level. Feedback should be requested from the learners, teachers and the leadership on the strengths and weaknesses of the remediation program. Consider conducting a morbidity and mortality assessment (M&M) model for each struggling learner

TABLE 12.2 Considerations for Creating Policies and Procedures

- Review institution's academic mission and philosophy
- Roles of remediation team members
- Resources to be utilized
- Competency-specific expectations/technical standards
- Identification, remediation, and reassessment methods
- Consequences of successful and failed remediation
- Address confidentiality vs. transparency
- Communication outside of remediation team
- Connection to promotions committee

to assess what worked and what did not work with that learner at your institution. The evolving literature, along with this feedback, should be used to continually modify and improve the program.

As either the program director or expert in remediation, it will be your responsibility to provide ongoing education for faculty. Unless your faculty have had a lot of experience with remediation, chances are you will have to teach them methods for educating and engaging struggling learners. There are 2 separate audiences for faculty education. All faculty need to be notified of the remediation program, its mission and philosophy and how to access the program when they identify a learner in need. This can occur through grand rounds presentations, presentations at committee meetings, faculty development workshops and online modules, such as those available through the University of Colorado School of Medicine Academy of Medical Educators website. (http://www.ucdenver.edu/academics/colleges/medicalschool/education/academy/Pages/default.aspx)

The second group of faculty is made up of your core remediation specialists. This group will need to be educated as all faculty, but will also need training on the diagnosis of learner deficits and the development of remediation plans. They should also be available to provide support for each other in discussing complicated or challenging cases and to learn from each other's experiences. Ideally, the core remediation specialists will have various clinical backgrounds and experience to provide a wealth of faculty expertise, which can be accessed depending on the primary diagnosed deficit. Depending on the need of your program, the specialists may each need up to 5% FTE to remediate a few learners per year.

Measurable outcomes to determine success

As briefly aforementioned, spend time upfront considering how you will determine the success of your program. A conversation should be scheduled with the leadership supporting you and the individuals and committees funding the program. How should success be measured? What is success? Is it the completion of the academic course, year or program? Is it better patient outcomes and decreased institutional risk? Is it learner satisfaction with the program? Is it student body satisfaction with the mission of your institution to see that all learners reach their maximum potential? Is it success if you mentor a learner towards an area of medicine more suited to their skills, even if that means not successfully completing your program? Does it mean encouraging an unsafe or unmotivated clinician to find a new career? They are all successes if you put the needs of the learner and patients as your priority. If 5% of your learners fail or leave the program, will your supporters see that as a success or mark your program as having failed? Perhaps success is having documentation that your learner was treated equally, fairly and was provided ample opportunities to demonstrate improvement.

Financial resources and institutional backing

The goal of any remediation program should be to assist the 15% of learners that are known to struggle; however, due to limits of time, faculty, and financial resources, a more practical goal may be the bottom 5 to 10% of every class. Given these limits, there is often debate as to who should provide the remediation: the department of the current rotation, the site of the current rotation or a larger entity. Since most deficits span several rotations or are identified (unfortunately) at the end of a rotation, the responsibility seems to fall on Student Affairs, the program director or institution.

- Consider the possible financial costs of the program:
- The remediation program director (FTE 20 to 50%)
- The core group of remediation specialists (FTE<5%)
- Administrative assistance
- Additional FTE support for institutional leaders, such as the Dean of Student Affairs
- Standardized patients, simulation and lab fees
- Video recordings
- Written examinations, question banks
- Web-based tools
- Clinical skills examinations
- Practice procedural equipment
- Psychiatric services
- Additional rotations beyond standard training
- Research assistance

While national medical education organizations have strongly supported remediation of learners, leadership at your institution may need to better understand its importance. Some institutions are less inclined or able to devote concentrated resources to a small number of learners. Other institutions feel that it is their educational mission and moral obligation. Clearly the more support the better. Where might resistance to the program come from? How can your program meet shared goals? What local barriers do you anticipate? Can you pilot the program? Also consider this: if your program is successful, how will your institution respond to your publications which acknowledge that you (like all institutions) have struggling learners?

Institutional support is also required to support faculty development initiatives in this area and to provide faculty time to dedicate to the cause. They may not be able to see as many patients while working directly with learners in remediation. They may need more non-clinical time to spend directly teaching and giving feedback to their learners.

Legal concerns

Program directors and administrative leadership, fearing the stress and financial burden of legal repercussions, may be reluctant to implement remediation plans, especially those that include probation, contract non-renewal, extension of training or dismissal. So I want to spend some time addressing the issue. In the US Supreme Court, the Regents of the University of Michigan v. Scott Ewing applied the principle of judicial nonintervention in academic decisions. Given the academic environment and need for qualified opinions, the courts have consistently upheld the rights of faculty, programs and institutions to make necessary disciplinary and remediation decisions for learners who are failing to progress academically.

For due process, the learner must be notified of her/his deficiency(ies) and its consequences. The learner must be given a chance to review the concerns and respond. The decisions made regarding disciplinary or remediation decisions must not be arbitrary.

While the fear of legal repercussion outweighs the actual risk, be sure to maintain complete documentation of the process from identification, to the leadership involved, the remediation plan instituted, how well it was followed and the outcomes measured. Of note, residency programs have been sued for graduating unfit or incompetent physicians. To the best of my knowledge, medical schools have not.

CHAPTER 13:

Outcomes Data

How many times have you heard or thought, "This learner should never become a doctor"? Yet s/he passed the clerkship or rotation or, more frightening, graduated without remediation. Medicine is a self-regulated profession and it is our responsibility to teach and monitor our own graduates. Take a moment to consider changes at your institution so that an incompetent learner will never graduate again.

Learners are worth investing in! There are many remediation success stories. Here are the outcomes from the University of Colorado Program from 2006–2011 (see **Figure 13.1**).

As you can see, not all learners succeeded to graduation or were returned to good academic standing. Some of the learners withdrew, were terminated, transferred or remain on probation.

Perhaps, it is worth mentioning when to stop remediation, i.e., when enough is enough.

1. The learner is working at her/his fullest capacity and not making significant progress. This assumes that a thorough investigation has discovered and attempted to treat all possible causes of her/his poor performance.
2. The learner is not invested in her/his remediation, despite multiple attempts to get her/him on board and address her/his individual barriers. Are you losing more nights of sleep worrying than your learner and spending more time trying to help the learner than they are willing to invest?
3. The learner is non-compliant with treatment of a severe psychiatric disorder or substance abuse or has a mental health or physical health problem that makes them unfit for duty (i.e. psychosis or seizures with stress or fatigue or accruing too many absences to be reliable or to learn).
4. The learner has timed out. How many years is the institution or program willing to invest and how much debt is the learner willing to accrue before remediation is futile? (e.g., failed USMLE Steps 3 times or more and therefore had training delayed, repeated more than 2 years of medical school, repeated more than 1 year of residency)

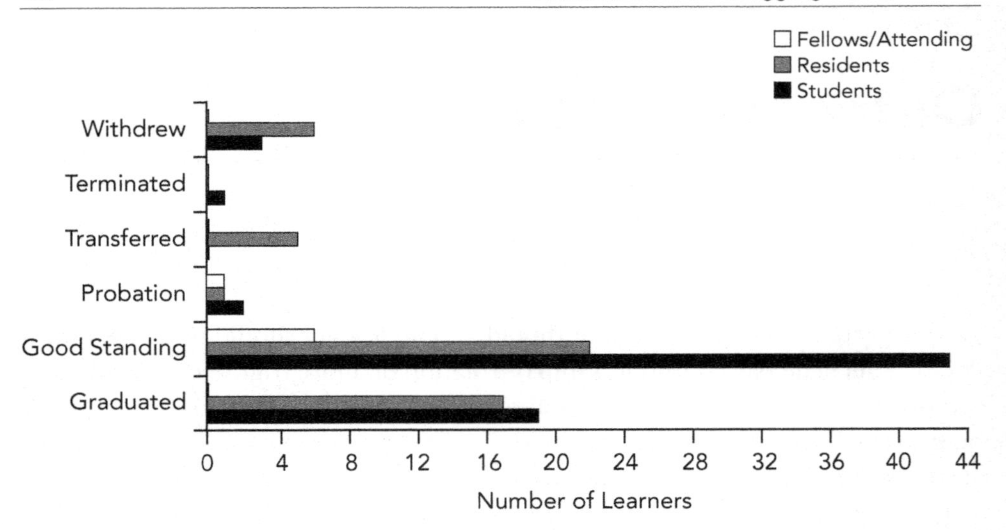

FIGURE 13.1 Performance Outcomes for Students and Residents Undergoing Remediation. Good standing refers to a learner who is actively enrolled without a letter of warning or probation. Transferred includes transfer of specialties, transfer to other programs of the same discipline or a switch to a research career/non-clinical career.

Let's take a look at some of the other data collected on the program (see **Figure 13.2**).

Feedback via survey was requested of all participants of the University of Colorado Program. Please see the learners' responses to the questions below.

When asked in what ways this program was helpful, written comments included:

- Helpful, honest timely feedback
- Specific guidelines and expectations
- Supportive and approachable faculty
- Recognition of improvement
- Customized to the learner's needs
- Improved confidence
- Extra teaching

When asked how can the program be improved in the future, written comments included:

- Not needed
- Improve learner honesty with the program

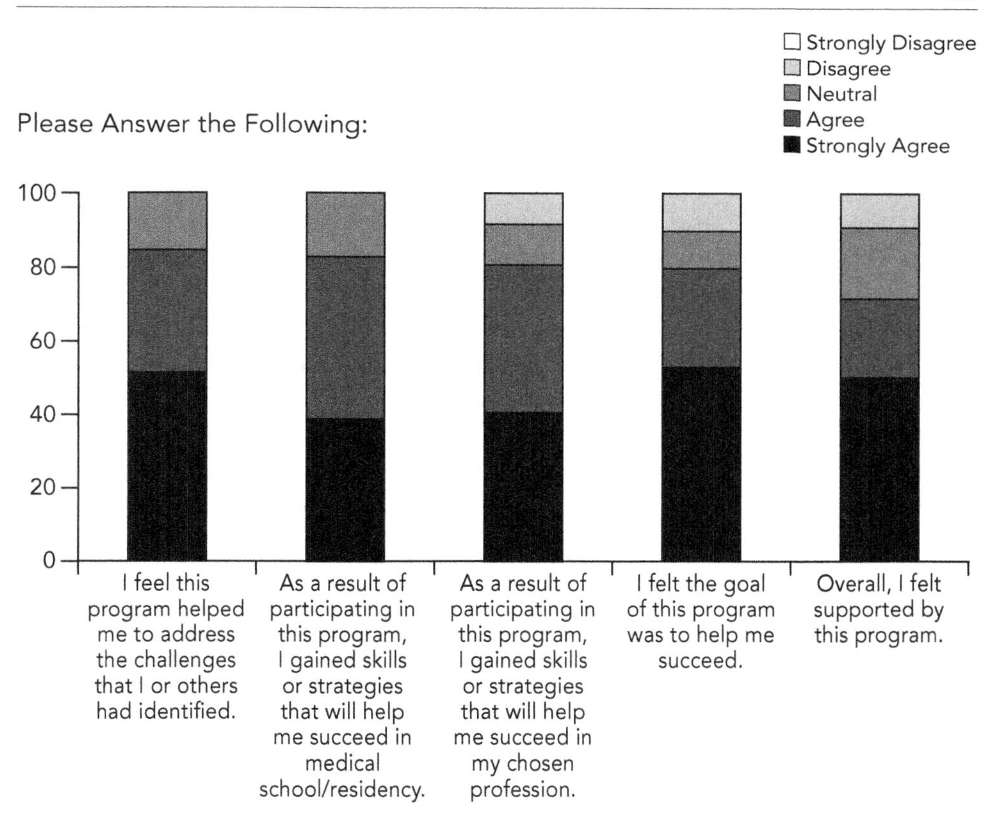

FIGURE 13.2 Voluntary Post-Remediation Feedback Survey Results, by Percent Response

- Need to be told directly that they will make it
- Knowing more about the program in advance
- Getting better feedback prior to having to remediate
- Cut down on clinical responsibilities during the remediation process

The challenge of struggling medical learners exists in all programs and they will continue to test the quality and flexibility of our programs and the teaching abilities of our faculty for decades to come. Can we individualize teaching effectively when it is most needed? We have a professional responsibility to our patients, community and professional colleagues to ensure that only competent learners graduate and remain in the practice of clinical medicine. The process of remediation cannot even begin without faculty and colleagues who are invested and feel ethically obligated to report the performance of underachieving learners. Don't get caught in the pitfalls. Encourage your colleagues to document their observations and assessment honestly and accurately with examples. Compare your learner's performance with her/his expected level of training, using a model like RIME or Dreyfus. Then a remediation team or faculty member can start with the broad differential referred to as ACGME Competencies "Plus" and collect additional information as needed to diagnose and confirm all of the learner's deficits. From there, the ONE greatest deficit can be selected on which to build a customized remediation plan.

It just takes a program leader and one or two faculty members to create a remediation program and another to perform blinded reassessment for success. Now you have algorithms to help guide you in your remediation efforts and suggestions for reassessment. Remember: deliberate practice, feedback and self-assessment are the key overarching principles of your remediation strategy!

You now know how to give effective feedback. In addition, you have read and practiced numerous cases that only add to your wealth of life experiences with weaker learners. You are more than prepared to begin helping those learners who need you most (even if your institution does not have a remediation program in place yet)!

If you have ever worked with a colleague or learner who you would not want to take care of you or your family, or to whom you were afraid to sign out coverage of your patients, then take the initiative to build a new remediation program or improve upon the one that already exists at your institution. Following your learner's and program's outcomes will lead to surprising results and improved outcomes and perhaps even a few publications.

Sometimes it can be a long, arduous process. Respond to this call to action and hang in there! It is worth the investment as you watch your learner flourish and go on to contribute to medicine in a positive way.

References/Resources

"American Board of Internal Medicine Faculty Development Conference: Evaluation of learners, Effective Feedback and Systems Approach." Eric Holmboe, University of Colorado Denver 2008.

Artino AR. Dong T. DeZee KJ. Gilliland WR. Waechter DM. Cruess D. Durning SJ. "Achievement goal structures and self-regulated learning: Relationships and changes in medical school." *Acad Med* 2012;87(10):1375–1381.

Blankenburg R. Long M. Rosenbluth G. Marisco N. Johnstone N. Dunagan M. Pantaleoni J. Augustine E. Stuart E. "Revisiting how we think: Innovative ideas for promoting and assessing clinical reasoning." *PAS* May 2011.

Boehler ML. "An investigation of medical student reactions to feedback: a randomized controlled trial." *Med Educ* 2006;40(8):746–9.

Carraccio CL. Benson BJ. Nixon LJ. Derstine PL. "From the educational bench to the clinical bedside: translating the Dreyfus developmental model to the learning of clinical skills." *Acad Med* 2008; 83(8):761–7.

Cleland J. Arnold R. Chessar A. "Failing finals is often a surprise for the student but not the teacher: identifying difficulties and supporting students with academic difficulties." *Med Teach* 2005;27(6):504–8.

DesRoches CM. Rao SR. Fromson JA. Birnbaum RJ. Iezzoni L. Vogeli C. Campbell E. "Physicians' perception, preparedness for reporting, and experiences related to impaired and incompetent colleagues." *JAMA* 2010; 304(2) 187–193.

Dudek NL. Marks MB. Regehr G. "Failure to fail: The perspectives of clinical supervisors." *Acad Med* 2005;80(10S):S84–7.

Eva KW. Rosenfeld J. Reiter HI. Norman GR. "An admissions OSCE: the multiple mini-interview." *Med Educ* 2004; 38(3):314–26.

Glanz K. Rimer BK. *Theory at a Glance: A Guide for Health Promotions Practice* 2nd ed. Washington D.C.: Department of Health and Human Services; 2005.

Guerrasio J. Cumbler EU. Trosterman A. Brandenburg SL. Wald HL. Aagaard EM. Can post-rotation evaluations detect residents in need of remediation? JGME 2012;3:47–51.

Guerrasio J. Garrity MJ. Aagaard EM. "Medical students, residents and attendings referred for remediation: Descriptive statistics and outcomes" Submitted.

Hauer KE. Ciccone A. Henzel TR. Katsufrakis P. Miller SH. Norcross WA. Papadakis MA. Irby DM. "Remediation of the deficiencies of physicians across the continuum from medical school to practice: a thematic review of the literature." *Acad Med* 2009; 84(12):1822–32.

Hodges B. Regehr G. Martin D. "Difficulties in recognizing one's own incompetence: novice physicians who are unskilled and unaware of it." *Acad Med* 2001;76(10):S87–89.

Holmboe ES. Yepes M. Williams F. Huot SJ. "Feedback and the mini clinical evaluation exercise." *JGIM* 2004;19(5pt2):558–61.

Hughes PH. Baldwin DC. Sheehan DV. Conard S. Storr CL. "Resident physician substance use, by specialty." *Am J Psychiatry* 1992; 149(10):1348–54.

Irby DM. Milam S. "The legal context for evaluating and dismissing medical students and residents." *Acad Med* 1989;64:639–643.

Kern DE, Thomas PA, Hughes MT. *Curriculum Development for Medical Education.* 2nd ed. Baltimore: The Johns Hopkins University Press. 2009.

Locke EA. "Motivation through conscious goal setting." *App Prevent Psych* 1996;5(2):117–124.

Malik S. "Students, tutors, and relationships: the ingredients of a successful support scheme." *Med Educ* 2000;34:635–641.

Neher JO. Stevens NG "The one-minute preceptor: shaping the teaching conversation." *Fam Med* 1992; 35(6):391–3.

Olmesdahl PJ. "The establishment of student needs: an important internal factor affecting course outcome." *Med Teach* 1999;21:174–9.

Oreskovich MR. Kaups KL. Balch CM. Hanks JB. Satele D. Sloan J. Meredith C. Budl A. Dyrbye LN, Shanafelt TD. "Prevalence of Alcohol Use Disorder Among American Surgeons." *Arch Surg* 2012;147(2):168–174.

The Outcomes Project. Accreditation Council for Graduate Medical Education. (www.acgme.org/outcome/comp/compFull.asp) 1999. Accessed December 15, 2012.

Pangaro L. "A new vocabulary and other innovations for improving descriptive in-training evaluations." *Acad Med* 1999; 74(11):1203–7.

Papadakis MA, Teherani A, Banach MA, Knettler TR, Rattner SL, Stern DT et al. "Disciplinary action by medical boards and prior behavior in medical school." *N Engl J Med* 2005; 353:2673–82.

Paul G. Hinman G. Dottl S. Passon J. "Academic development: a survey of academic difficulties experiences by medical students and support services provided." *Teach Learn Med* 2009: 21(3):254–60.

"The problem resident" VHS videocassette produced by ABIM; 1992.

Reamy BV. Harman JH. "Residents in trouble: An in-depth assessment of the 25 year experience of a single family medicine residency." *Fam Med* 2006;38(4):252–257.

Rheum J. "Pygmalion in the classroom." *NTLF* 1999;8(2).

Saxena V. O'Sullivan PS. Teherani A. Irby DM. Hauer KE. "Remediation techniques for student performance problems after a comprehensive clinical skills assessment." *Acad Med* 2009; 84(5):669–676.

Saxon D. Boylan H. "The cost of remedial education in higher education." *J Develop Educ* 2001;25(2):2–8.

Schwind CJ. Williams RG, Boehler ML, Dunnington GL. "Do individual attendings' post rotation performance ratings detect residents' clinical performance deficiencies?" *Acad Med.* 2004:79;453–457.

Shapiro J. Prislin MD. Larsen KM. Lenahan PM. "Working with the resident in difficulty." *Fam Med* 1987:19:368–75.

Shute VJ. "Focus on formative feedback." *Rev Educ Res* 2008; 78(1),153–189.

Vaughn LM. Baker RC. Thomas DG. "The problem learner." *Teach Learn Med* 1998;10:217–22.

Wiese JG. "Strong as Our Weakest Link. Presentation." Tulane University Health Sciences Center. 2006.

Winter RO. "Working with impaired residents: trials, tribulations, and successes." *Fam Med* 2002;34(3):190–6.

Wolpaw TM. Wolpaw DR. Papp KK. "SNAPPS: a learner-centered model for outpatient education." *Acad Med* 2003;78(9):893–8.

Yao DC. Wright SM. "A national survey of internal medicine residency program directors regarding problem residents." *JAMA* 2000; 284;1099–104.

Yao DC. Wright SM. "The challenge of problem residents." *J Gen Intern Med* 2001;16:486–92.

Yates J. James D. "Predicting the strugglers: A case-control study of students at Nottingham University Medical School. *BMJ* 2006;332:1009–1013.

Recommended Resources

Journal Articles:

Aagaard EM. Teherani A. Irby D. "Effectiveness of the one-minute preceptor model for diagnosing the patient and the learner: Proof of concept." *Academic Medicine* 2004;79(1)42–9.

Berner ES, Graber ML. "Overconfidence as a cause of diagnostic error in medicine." *American Journal of Medicine* 2008;121(5suppl):S2–23.

Boiselle PM. "A remedy for resident evaluation and remediation." *Academic Radiology* 2005; 12:894–900.

Bordage G. "Conceptual frameworks to illuminate and magnify." *Medical Education* 2009;43:312–19.

Bordage G. "Why did I miss the diagnosis? Some cognitive explanations and educational implications." *Academic Medicine* 1999;74(10)S138–43.

Carraccio CL. Benson BJ. Nixon LJ. Derstine PL. "From the educational bench to the clinical bedside: translating the Dreyfus developmental model to the learning of clinical skills." *Academic Medicine* 2008; 83(8):761–7.

Ericsson KA. "Deliberate practice and the acquistition and maintenance of expert performance in medicine and related domains." *Academic Medicine* 2004;79(10):S70–81.

Eva KW. "What every teacher needs to know about clinical reasoning." *Medical Education* 2005;41:281–87.

Hauer KE. Ciccone A. Henzel TR. Katsufrakis P. Miller SH. Norcross WA. Papadakis MA. Irby DM. "Remediation of the deficiencies of physicians across the continuum from medical school to practice: a thematic review of the literature." *Academic Medicine* 2009; 84(12):1822–32.

Irby DM. "What clinical teachers in medicine need to know." *Academic Medicine* 1994;69(5)333–42.

Pangaro L. "A new vocabulary and other innovations for improving descriptive in-training evaluations." *Academic Medicine* 1999; 74(11):1203–7.

Saxena V. O'Sullivan PS. Teherani A. Irby DM. Hauer KE. "Remediation techniques for student performance problems after a comprehensive clinical skills assessment." *Academic Medicine* 2009; 84(5):669–676.

Winston KA. Van Der Vleuten CPM. Scherpbier AJJA. "An investigation into the design and effectiveness of a mandatory cognitive skills programme for at-risk medical students." *Medical Teacher* 2010;32:236–243.

Wolpaw TM. Wolpaw DR. Papp KK. "SNAPPS: a learner-centered model for outpatient education." *Academic Medicine* 2003;78(9):893–8.

Yao DC. Wright SM. "The challenge of problem residents." *Journal of General Internal Medicine* 2001;16:486–92.

Websites:

Competencies: www.acgme.org/outcome/comp/compHome.asp

Educational guidance: www.aamc.org

Faculty Development: www.ucdenver.edu/academics/colleges/medicalschool/education/academy/Pages/default.aspx

Remediation information, webinars, events: www.clinicalremediation.com; www.jeannetteguerrasiomd.com

Texts:

Cooke M. Irby DM. O'Brien BC. *Educating Physicians.* San Francisco: Jossey-Bass, 2010.

Dhaliwal G. Clinical Decision-Making: Understanding How Clinicians Make Diagnoses. In Saint S. Crazen J. Solomon C. *NEJM Clinical Problem Solving.* (pp. 19–30). Boston: Massachusetts Medical Society, 2006.

Kassirer JP. Wong JB. Kopelman RI. *Learning Clinical Reasoning.* Philadelphia: Lippincott Williams & Wilkins, 2009.

Kern DE. Thomas PA. Hughes MT. *Curriculum Development for Medical Education.* 2nd ed. Baltimore: The Johns Hopkins University Press, 2009.

Other:

Pre-clinical and Clinical Learning Surveys, copyrighted by the President and Fellows of Harvard College 2010. These can be obtained by contacting Laurie W. Raymond, MD at laurie_raymond@hms.harvard.edu.

Learning Assessments at www.vark-learn.com.

Observation guide at www.skillscascade.com/handouts/CalgaryCambridgeGuide.pdf

Research Collaboration:

If you are interested in collaborating on multi-institution studies related to research on remediation, please e-mail: Jeannette.Guerrasio@ucdenver.edu.

ABOUT THE AUTHOR

Jeannette Guerrasio, MD

Jeannette Guerrasio, MD is currently an Associate Professor of Medicine at the University of Colorado, where she practices internal medicine as a hospitalist and has dedicated her academic career to working with struggling medical learners. While she was trained as a medical doctor and spends a majority of her time teaching medical students, residents, fellows, junior colleagues and occasionally nurse practitioners, her expertise in the remediation of medical learners bridges the professional medical community. At the University of Colorado, Dr. Guerrasio has built a unique and highly successful remediation program, which includes the development of individualized learning plans. She has lectured and led workshops at national, regional and local conferences and has developed a national reputation for her work and expertise in this area. In 2010, she was awarded the Excellence in Education Award for Mentoring and Advising by the Academy of Medical Educators, in 2011 was chosen by the graduating class as the best clinical teacher and in 2012 she was inducted in to the University of Colorado's Academy of Medical Educators.

Additional information about the author and upcoming events are available at www.clinicalremediation.com.

ABOUT THE

Association for Hospital Medical Education (AHME)

The Association for Hospital Medical Education, founded in 1956, is a national, nonprofit professional organization involved in the continuum of hospital-based medical education. AHME's members represent several hundred teaching hospitals, academic medical centers, and consortia which are involved in the delivery of undergraduate, graduate, and continuing medical education. The Mission of AHME is to: promote improvement in medical education to meet health care needs; serve as a forum and resource for medical education information; develop professionals in the field of medical education; and advocate the value of medical education in health care.

To fulfill its Mission, the Association annually provides: a three-day educational conference (AHME Institute); several one-day educational sessions (AHME Academy); a series of six teleconferences; the AHME *Guide to Medical Education in the Teaching Hospital* (a practical, 425-page resource for medical education professionals); two issues of *AHME News*; as well as additional resources on its website (www.ahme.org). AHME secures external funding to support clinical performance-improvement activities, solicits and reviews proposals from member institutions, and awards grants to support these projects. AHME publishes the *Journal for Continuing Education in the Health Professions*, a peer-reviewed publication, in collaboration with the Alliance for Continuing Education in the Health Professions (ACEHP) and the Society of Academic Continuing Medical Education (SACME). The Association also co-sponsors the quadrennial CME Congress with ACEHP, SACME, and the Canadian Association for Continuing Health Education.

AHME supports four interest groups which include: the Council of Administrative Directors of Medical Education; the Council on Continuing Medical Education; the Council of Program Administrators and Coordinators; and the Council of Transitional Year Program Directors. The Association is a member organization of the Accreditation Council for Continuing Medical Education and the Education Commission for Foreign Medical Graduates, as well as an associate member organization of the Council of Medical Specialty Societies. It also enjoys collaborative relationships with a number of other accreditation, regulatory, and professional organizations with an interest in medical education.

Index

CPSIA information can be obtained
at www.ICGtesting.com
Printed in the USA
BVOW06s2051190617
487049BV00025B/269/P